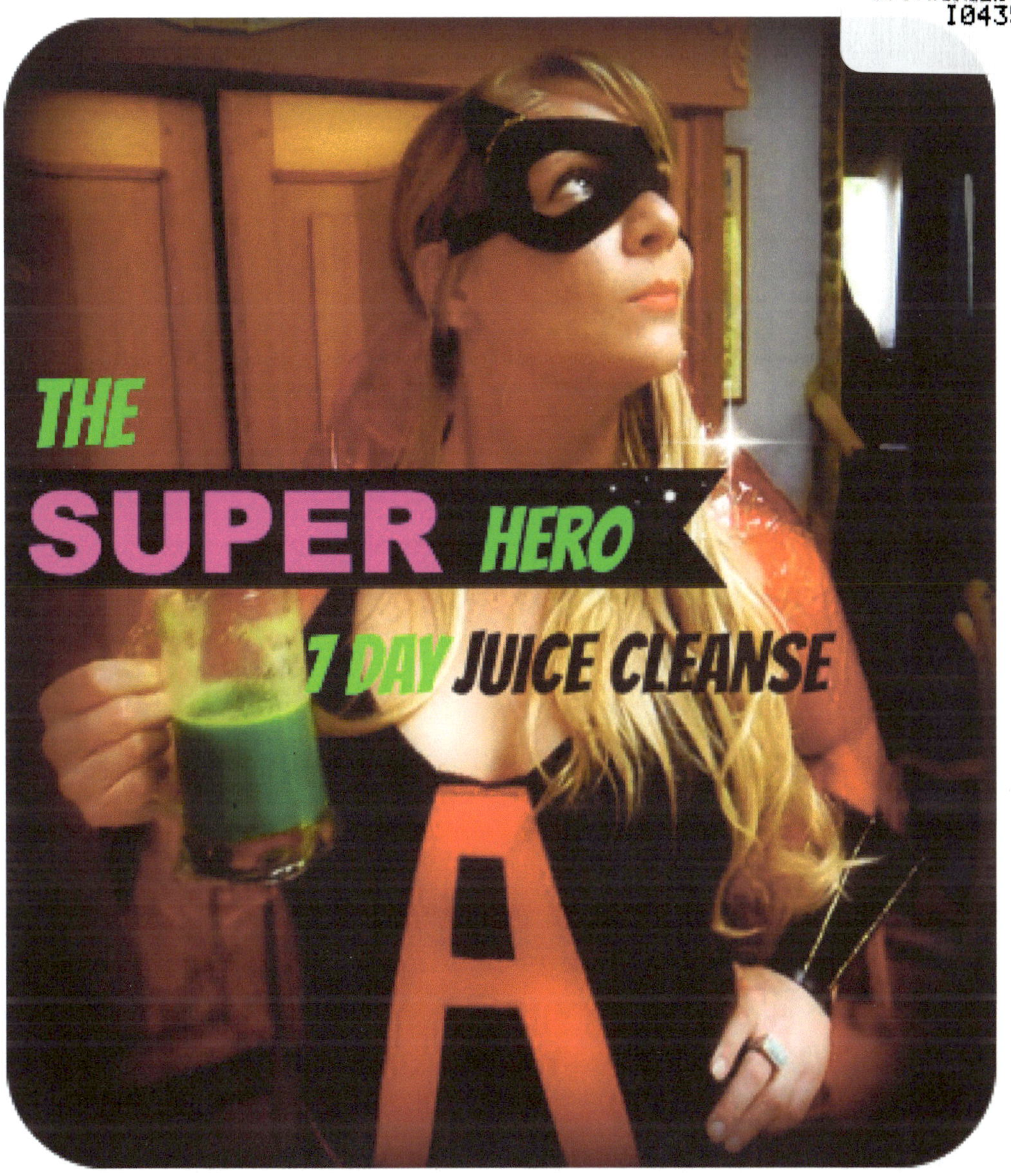

THE SUPER HERO
7 DAY JUICE CLEANSE

GO ON, BE A SUPER HERO!

WITH SUPER LOVE,

Emyrald Sinclaire

1

WHAT OTHER SUPER HEROES ARE SAYING....

DAWN BROWNING, PH. D., NEW MEXICO – ""The Superhero Juice Cleanse was

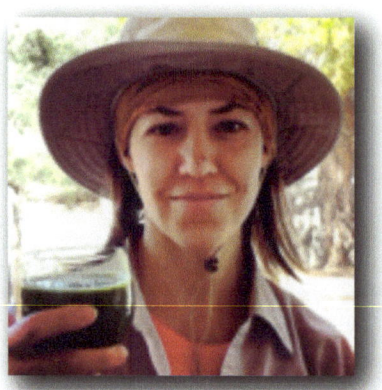 **exceptionally well-orchestrated**. In addition to relevant background material and **EXCELLENT juice and soup recipes**, Emyrald incorporates critical components of any good cleanse that others often lack: **yoga, affirmations, exercise, and moral support**. I emerged from this cleanse with tremendous **mental clarity, a glowing complexion, a lightness of being,** and most importantly – an **enhanced awareness of how my body functions** and what it needs. It is a great cleanse!"

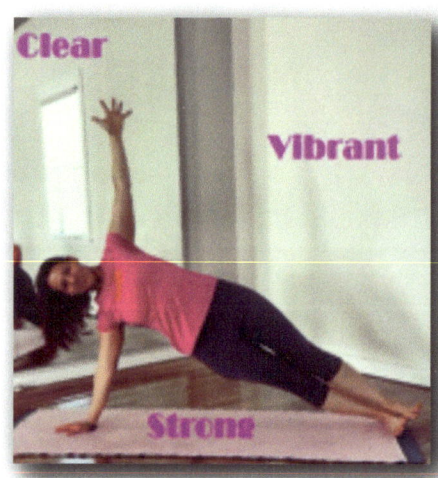

KIM BOWEN, PROSPER WELLNESS AZ– "I'll be honest, I really didn't think I

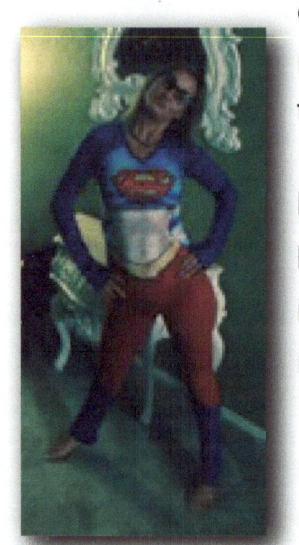 could do 7 days of juicing, but it was easy once I got going and now I continue to mostly juice during the day & have a meal in the evening because I feel so good!

I **lost pounds**, have **less cellulite**, and **plenty more energy**! But the big one for me is **NO MORE SUGAR CRAVINGS**. Just do it. All the info you need, Emyrald has provided. PLUS I feel even more like a **Super Woman**!" www.ProsperWellnessAZ.com

Inside of This SUPER AWESOME Book You'll Find:

A Few More Words of Inspiration before we begin:

Jen Varriano, Inspiring Om– "I just completed the 7 Day Juice cleanse…

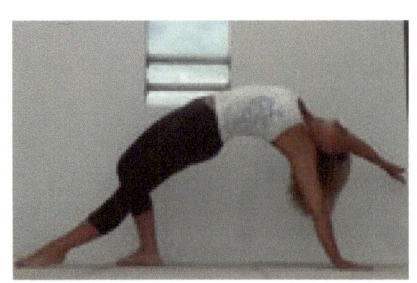

drinking fresh pressed juices to cleanse the body and mind. I already know the many benefits of juice cleansing, and I am a pretty good judge as to when my body is ready to play and when it needs to get down and dirty… this playful cleanse enabled me to do both… and reap personal rewards… **identifying my personal Super Powers!** Now to check my list of super powers, one by one:

#1: I believe I could Fly and Run faster than a Speeding Bullet!
#2: I could See through Walls with the power of Discernment!
#3: My Killer Kiss has Activated Taste Buds.
#4: I could just about Predict the Future as it relates to my gut.
#5: My Skin Glows.
#6: I have the ability to Stretch into Any Imaginable Form.

If you are considering a cleanse and are ready to take your life to **SuperHero status**… an experienced cleanser can take you there!" www.InspiringOm.com

Amber, Illinois – "I loved doing this 7 day juice cleanse! There were days I didn't know if I could make it through, but I'm so glad I stuck with it! By the end of the week I had so much more energy and just felt so much better overall. I also lost some weight over the week, which made me feel better in my clothes as well. I definitely plan on repeating this cleanse many more times to come and would highly recommend it!"

Zach, Illinois – "There were ups and downs doing the juice cleanse, but I was happy that I finished the week. The recipes were very good and the soups were amazing! I felt much better at the end of the week and had more energy than I anticipated. I will be doing the cleanse again for sure."

A Personal Note from A Juicing SUPERhero…

I bet secretly – deep down inside – you've always thought of yourself as a Superhero, am I correct? Knowing that you're prepared – you've got your 'gear' on below your work clothes and glasses ready to be tossed off for when the world needs saving, yes?

For all of us that secretly (or not so secretly) have a mask, boots, and cape on 'stand-by' for when the moment calls, then this book is for you!!

And if you're a little bit shy to embrace your **AMAZING, SUPER, POWERFUL, RADIANT, SUPER-HERO** side, then allow this book to be your inspiration to allow that superhero hiding inside to burst out!!

I mean it when I say it.....Go on, Be a Superhero!

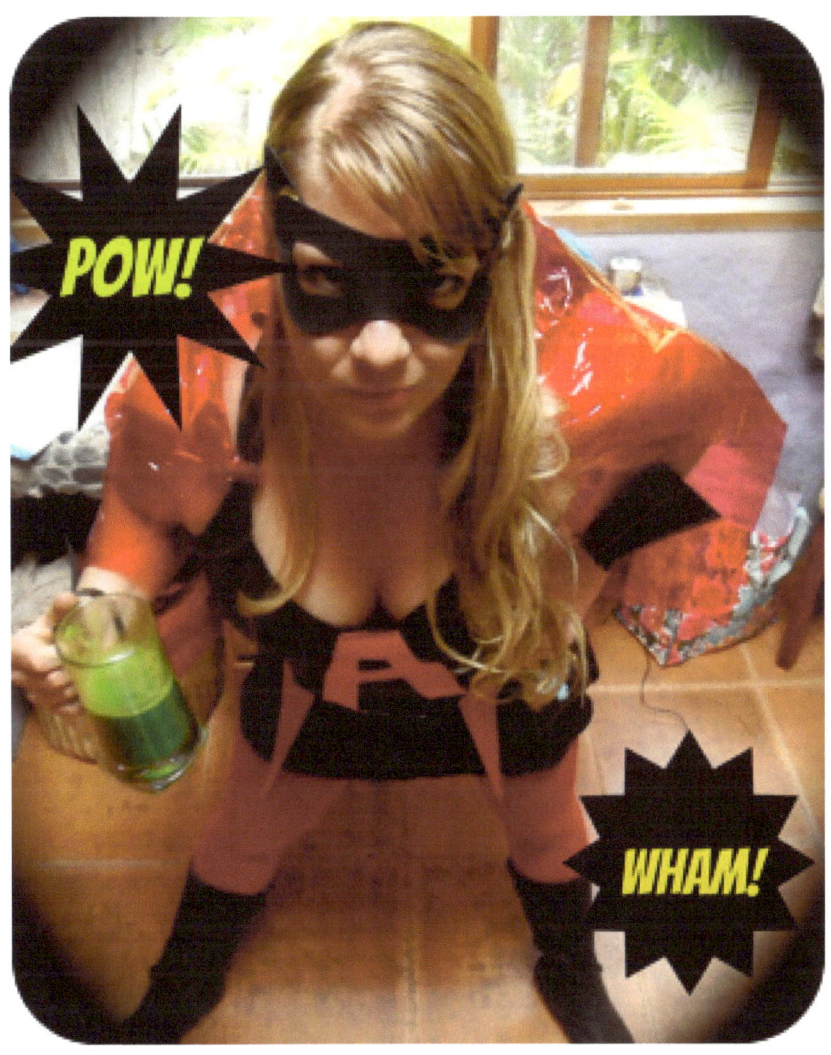

THE IMPORTANCE OF DETOXIFICATION & CLEANSING

First of all, I want to say **"Congratulations"** for picking up this book. Something has inspired you to start or continue your juicing journey and I'm already so very proud of you!

Did you know that we use about 70% of our available energy for digestion? Now, imagine if that energy was freed up to be put to other uses such as: **breaking down cancerous tissues, eliminating heavy metals from the body, removing toxins and pesticides from fat cells, and many more healing purposes**. When we remove the task of digestion, by consuming only pure, ORGANIC, fiberless fruit and vegetable juice, we have so much more energy to heal our bodies!

Not only that, once we clear the crud out of our bodies, our minds are much more clear. Our intuition develops. Answers to problems become clearer. Life seems brighter. We sleep better. We make better decisions because we see issues from more angles. As a result, our interpersonal relationships improve.

A LITTLE BIT OF BACKGROUND INFORMATION ON YOUR CELLS...

Energy comes from the little powerhouses in the body called cells of which there are over 75 trillion, right now all working together to produce the living breathing you. In these cells all the nutrients from our food are processed, the waste eliminated and energy is produced. So in looking at health and what constitutes the best food for us to eat we need to look at exactly what it is that causes our cells not only to survive, but more importantly, to thrive. To find the ultimate recipe for health we need to break down what it is that every cell in our body needs to thrive.

WHAT HEALTHY CELLS NEED:
1. Oxygen
2. Nutrients
3. The ability to detoxify

It makes sense that in order to **maximize our overall health, maintain our optimal weigh**t and **assist in reversing or preventing aging and disease** we must maximize the functionality and efficiency of each of the cells in our body.

One of the easiest and most efficient ways to positively impact your health is through the food choices you make. Many studies have shown that proper nutrition ALWAYS plays a central role in disease prevention and the restoration of health! Study after study shows a wealth of evidence to support the fact that **our diets can nourish as well as heal us. Behold the power of food**!!

Whole food nutrition allows the body to use its built-in restorative ability and will assist the body's capacity to heal itself. Or in this case, **juicing**!

DETOXIFICATION OF THE BODY...

Detoxification is a normal process within the body as it neutralizes and eliminates toxins through the major organs, such as our **colon, liver, kidneys, lungs, lymph nodes and skin**. Our bodies do it naturally every day, in fact it is one of our most basic automatic functions. But **what if our self-cleaning system is overloaded by our unhealthy lifestyle and exposure to environmental toxins?**

According to many healing experts, detoxification through special cleansing programs such as juicing may be **the missing link to disease prevention,** especially for immune-deficiency diseases like cancer, arthritis, diabetes, chronic fatigue syndrome and candida. Our chemical-laden diet, with an overabundance of animal protein, too much saturated fat, too much sugar and too much caffeine and alcohol radically alters our internal ecosystem. However, even if your diet is good, we still live in a dirty world. A cleanse can restore your immune system and protect yourself against environmental toxins that pave the way for disease bearing bacteria, viruses and parasites.

ONE THING TO CONSIDER...

You may become an emotional mess! It's no fun but it's true. When you are juice cleansing, stored emotions arise for the body to release. This can result in angry outbursts, fits of tears, extreme fatigue and so much more.

Not to worry. Anything and everything you experience is completely normal. We all experience detoxification differently. Just be with the process. Laugh and smile and if you need to, retreat to the privacy of a good book if you can. Take these seven days to get in touch with your body and mind and emotional state. Try to clear your calendar and look after yourself as much as possible. Keep any

distractions to a minimum. This includes TV, business appointments, and anything else that might divide your attention.

To get the most out of the cleanse, it's important that you are in a supportive environment and remain in a relaxed state. And at the same time, I understand that we are all very busy individuals. This 7-day cleanse is built to fit into any lifestyle.

So if the only thing you can change is the fact that you are adding juices to your daily diet, then...

THAT IS PERFECT!

THAT IS FANTASTIC!

THAT IS AMAZING!

I already think you are a SUPERhero for taking this first step!

SuperMom agrees and says:

"Don't make me spank you with my wooden spoon! Go on, be a SUPERhero today!"

Trust me, you don't want to make SuperMom angry.

You best do what she says.

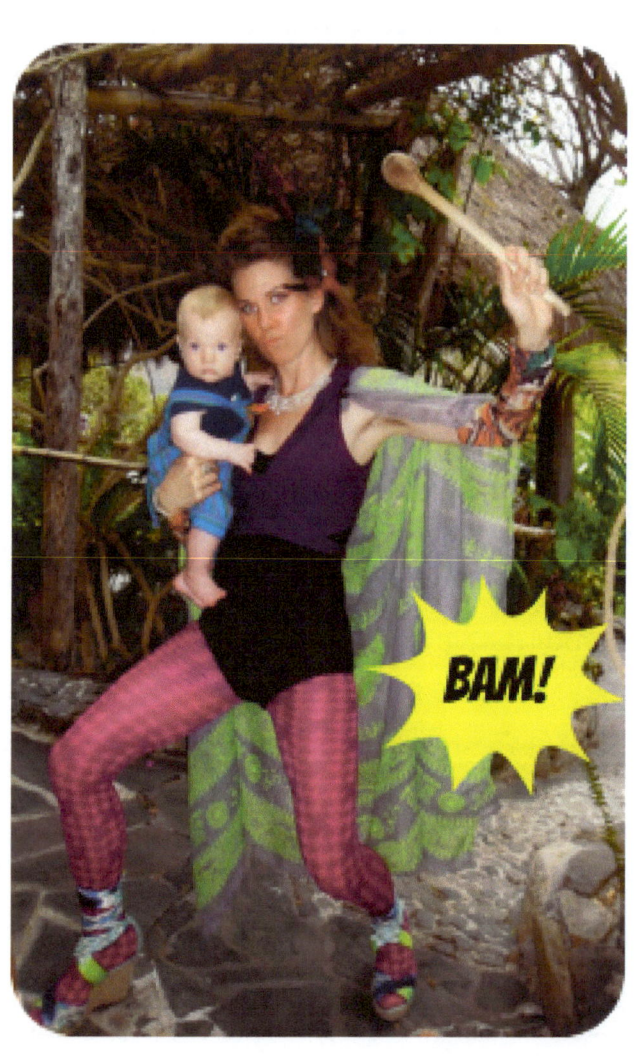

Juices versus Smoothies

Do you know the difference between a juice and a smoothie? Many people get confused, it's okay. I'll wave my magic wand and give you the answer faster than the speed of light!! (Ok, maybe not really at lightning speed, but I will clear things up for you.)

A Juice

A juicer separates the fibrous pulp of vegetables (and harder fruits) from the liquid, which contains all the vitamins and minerals; this is called a juice. Most juicers can easily juice a variety of harder fruits and vegetables including (but definitely not limited to): kale, cucumbers, carrots, celery, beets, ginger, garlic, radishes, swiss chard, bok choy, broccoli, sweet potatoes, and apples.

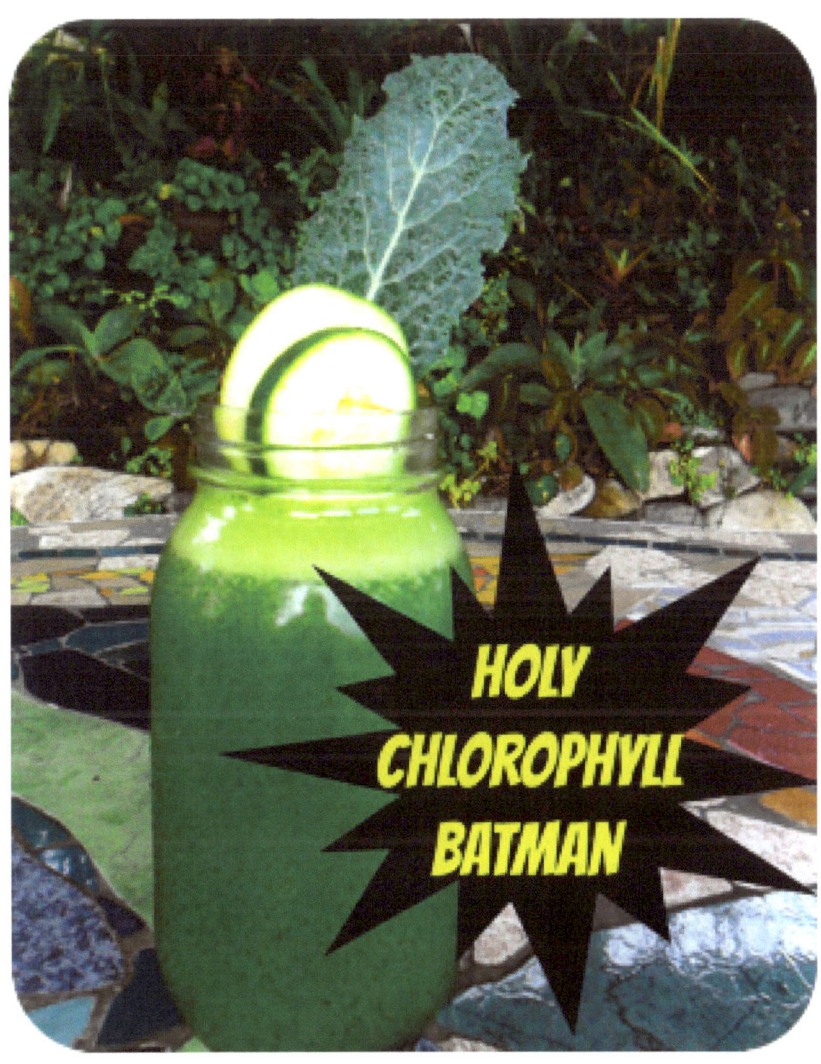

There are a variety of juicer types* on the market that operate in slightly different fashions from each other. But the result is the same: pure vitamins and minerals extracted from the vegetables in liquid form that is easily absorbed straight into the blood stream.

Sound too good to be true!? It's not. It's something straight out of a magic show right there. A magic show in your kitchen!

*https://www.youtube.com/watch?v=jifTvPYeRP0

SMOOTHIES

A quick and easy explanation about smoothies:

CHOP UP SOME FRUITS AND VEGGIES, THROW THEM IN THE BLENDER WITH SOME LIQUID AND BLEND ON HIGH.

Viola! That's a smoothie. The fiber and the liquid stay together in one juicy package.

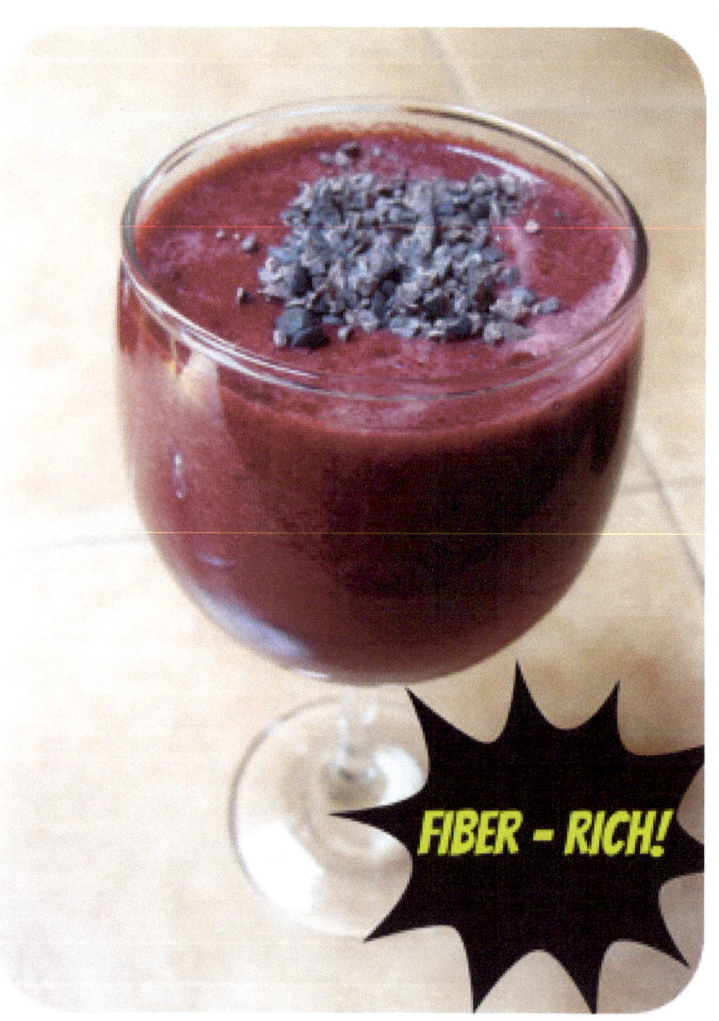

FIBER - RICH!

We won't be making smoothies in this Superhero cleanse. But that's not to say they are a bad thing. I LOVE smoothies. They are fantastic for many reasons. But for sake of argument and for sake of time ₍who's going to save the planet if we're both sitting here reading for pages and pages?₎, move beyond your thoughts of:

"HOLY RED SMOOTHIE, WONDER WOMAN, THAT LOOKS TASTY!"

And get back into your Juicing Mentality.

Thanks.

THE BENEFITS OF JUICING

Books have been written on the benefits of juicing. However, I will simply give you the basic outline. You're smart, you're a **SUPERhero** – you get the idea.

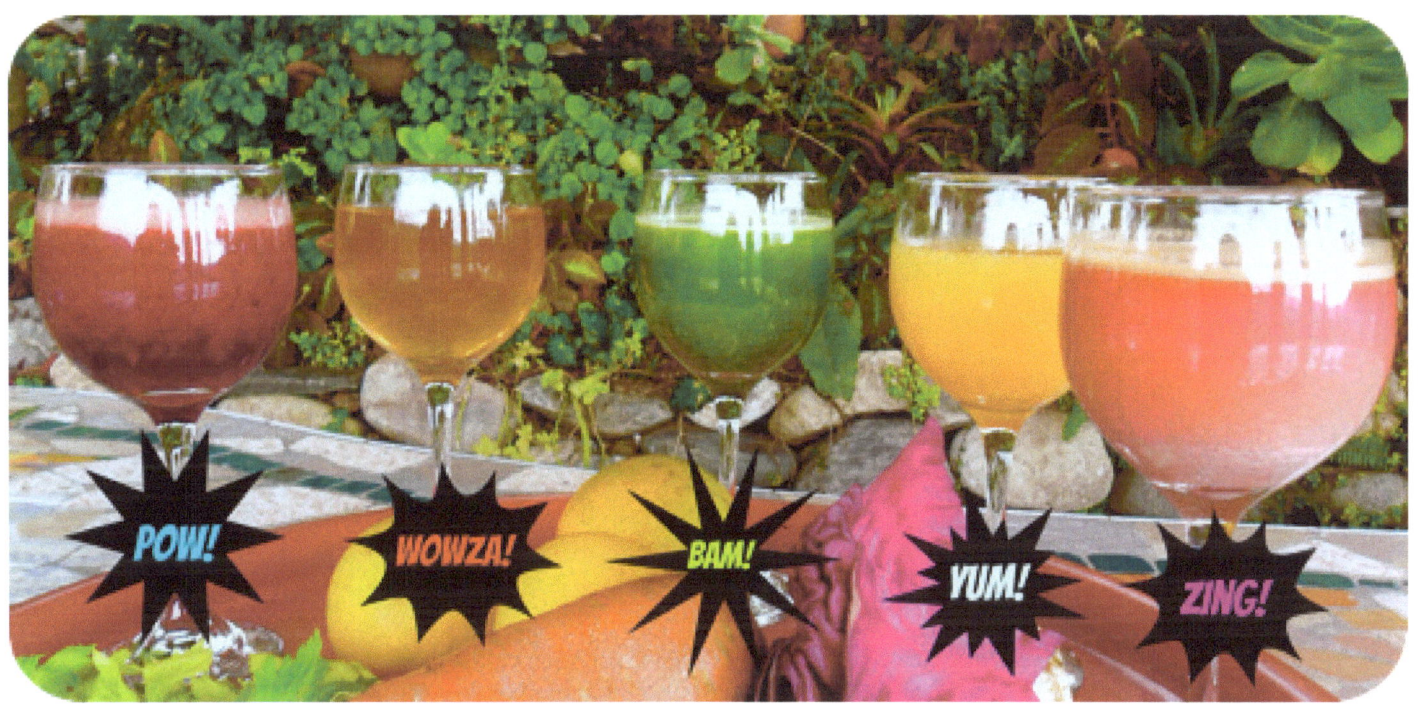

1. HIGH VITAMIN AND MINERAL CONTENT

When you juice a fruit or vegetable, you drink the liquid form of all the vitamins and minerals, which then goes immediately into the bloodstream and body systems. Fresh juice nourishes your body with vitamin rich and easy to digest nutrition.

2. DETOXIFYING FOR THE BODY

Fresh juices are full of the vitamins and minerals that our bodies require that we sometimes don't get. When our bodies are satisfied in their need of proper nutrients, energy is freed up to cleanse the body of trapped toxins. This can also lead to weight-loss, more energy and a better overall mentality.

3. YOUTHFUL ENERGY AND APPEARANCE

When you load up on all the antioxidants, vitamins, and minerals in a concentrated cup or two daily, it helps to fight wrinkles, eliminate free radicals, and add moisture and a glow to your skin.

4. WEIGHT-LOSS

Juicing helps us to maintain (or get to) our normal body weight. When we give our bodies the nutrients it needs, it can easily get to homeostasis (equilibrium in the systems of the body). Juicing can take the place of high-calorie snacks and because there is so much nutrition in one glass of vegetable juice, many find that their cravings go away.

5. ADDING MISSING NUTRITION TO THE DIET

Juicing puts a larger variety of vegetables into your diet. We tend to get into a routine with our vegetable choices. But with juicing, you can get a much larger variety of vegetables into the diet leading to a wider variety of minerals and vitamins present in your body.

Additional vitamins and minerals help you to see through walls, jump over buildings in a single bound and to fly around the planet at least 10 times while reciting the alphabet…backwards.

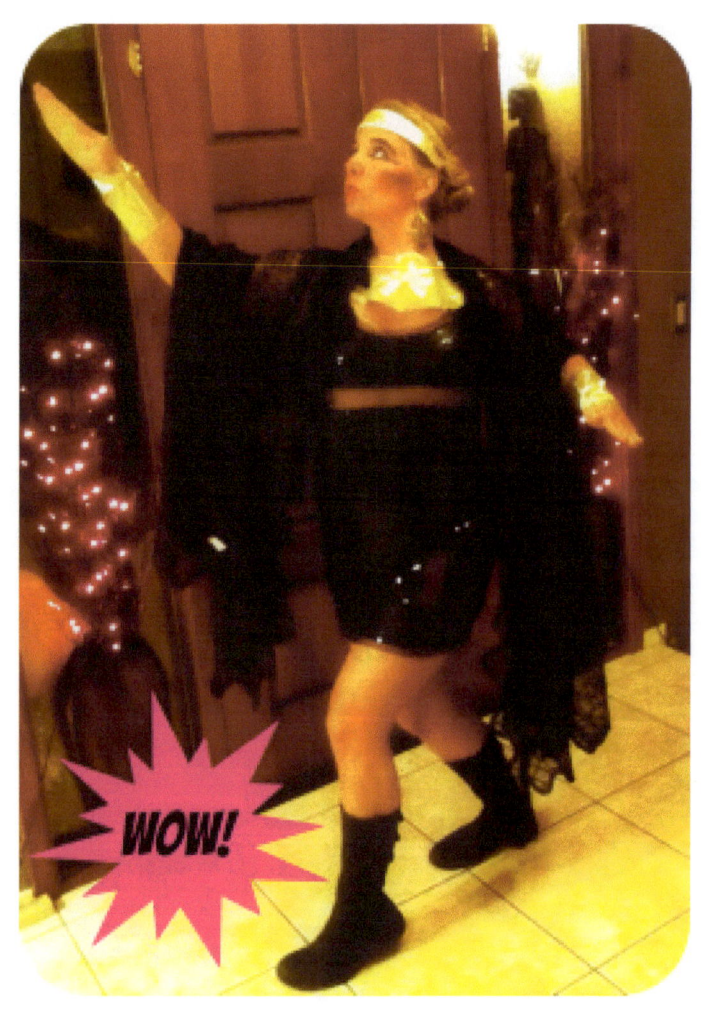

Comparisons between Juicers

There are many types of juicers on the market today and it can be quite confusing when you're bombarded with so many choices! I'm going to explain the three types of juicers to you so you can decide which one is the best for you!

Centrifugal

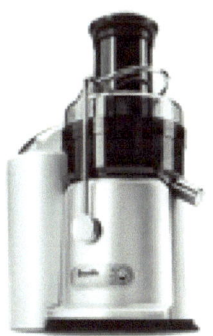

Centrifugal juicers are generally the most common and usually the most affordable. They typically have an upright design in which food is pushed into a rapidly spinning mesh chamber with sharp teeth on its floor. The teeth shred the food into a pulp, and the centrifugal motion pulls the juice out of the pulp and through the mesh filter, where it is funneled out of the juicer via a spigot. The pulp is filtered into a separate compartment.

Centrifugal juicers work best with soft and hard fruits and vegetables, but not quite as well with leafy greens like kale or spinach, or with wheatgrass.

Masticating

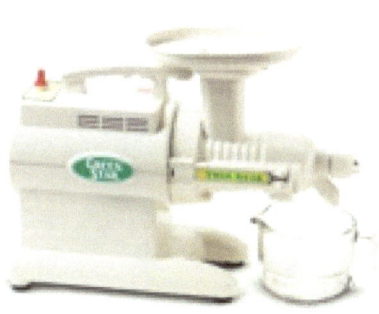

Masticating juicers typically have a horizontal design in which a tube containing the auger extends out of the motorized base. Pieces of fruits and vegetables are pushed into the top of the tube, and they are crushed and squeezed by the auger. Juice drains out of the underside of the tube, while the pulp is squeezed out at the end of the tube.

Because of the slower crushing and squeezing action, masticating juicers can process leafy greens and wheatgrass with ease but aren't so great with soft fruits and vegetables.

Slow Juicer/Upright Juicer

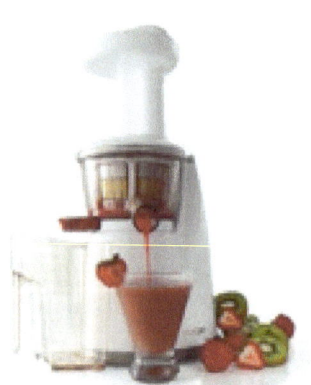

This type of juicer has an upright design similar to centrifugal juicers, but operates similar to the masticating juicer, with the auger or gear crushing the food and pressing out the juice.

Slow Juicers juice hard fruits and vegetables and leafy greens with ease, but its downside is softer fruits and vegetables.

So which one should you use?

You can use any juicer you like for this program. I own both a centrifugal and a slow juicer and use them both interchangeably depending on the type of juice I'm making that day.

If the juice calls for many leafy greens like kale and spinach, I like to juice them through the **slow juicer or the masticating**.

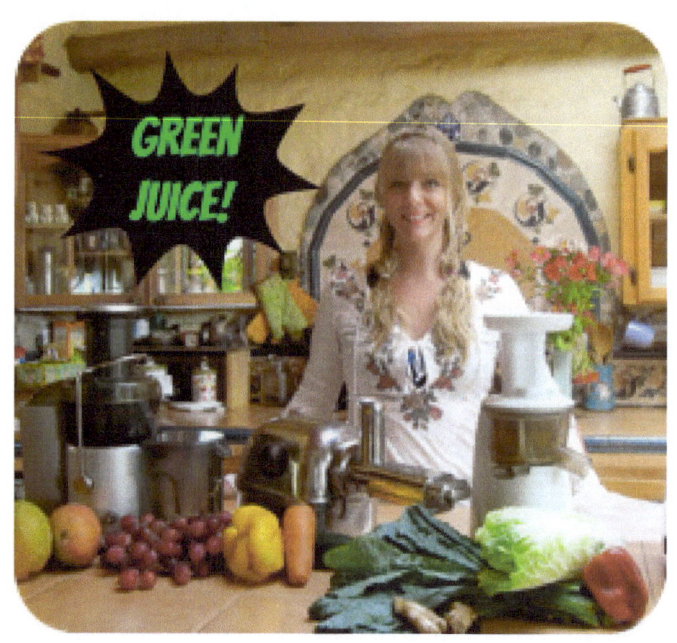

If the juice calls for plenty of harder vegetables such as carrots and cucumbers, I use the **centrifugal** because it's faster for that type of work.

For this cleanse, I think the slow or masticating juicers are better. But if you only have a centrifugal, that's just fine, too.

The most important part is to make juice!

7 Day Exercise Plan

Exercise and movement are a very important part of the cleansing process. They improve circulation and help expel toxins and relax the body. Daily exercise is a requirement to being healthy. **During this cleanse we will be exercising every single day for 30 non-stop minutes** (At a minimum. Feel free to exercise more if you desire). The key is to **get the heart rate up and to keep it there**.

I'm not going to tell you what exactly you should do as we all have different desires. The most important thing is that it is something you enjoy. Then it won't feel like exercise! Once again –the goal is at least **30 minutes a day every day**!

Exercise options include:
- Hiking
- Running
- Walking at a brisk pace
- Jogging
- Pushing a child in a stroller
- Cycling
- Touch-football
- Soccer

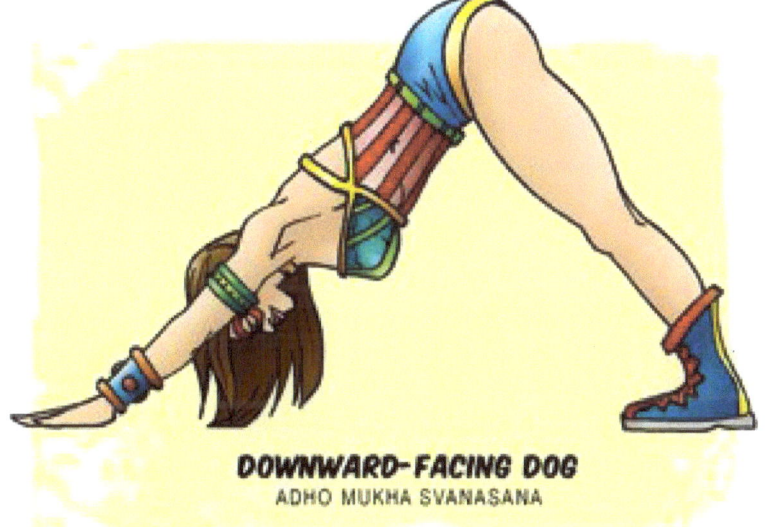

DOWNWARD-FACING DOG
ADHO MUKHA SVANASANA

Yoga

Daily yoga is important to keep the body and mind flexible. Not only that, the twisting and moving of the body helps to expel toxins from the body.

Once again, your goal will be 30 minutes (minimum) of yoga a day. Yoga is now so widely popular that you can find classes in almost any city at studios, gyms, recreation centers and more! And you can even find yoga classes online! My favorite websites include: **YogaGlo.com, MyYogaOnline.com,** and **DoYogaWithMe.com**. There are plenty more! Pick a style that suits your level and get your body moving!

Suggested Supplements & Herbs for Detox

There are a variety of plants that help support your cleansing organs, such as the liver, kidneys, bowels and skin. While these supplements and herbs are not REQUIRED for this cleanse, they are pretty darn fantastic and deserve to be mentioned because they are SUPERheroes in and of themselves! I suggest you try some of them out. If you like some, keep using them long after this cleanse. **We live in a dirty world and anything you can do to help your body get the toxins out, is a good thing**. These aren't **NECESSARY** to cleanse, just **SUGGESTED**. (You can find most of these products in your local health-food store or online at Amazon.com. Look for high-quality products without fillers.)

Ginger Lemon Detox Tea

Ginger is a powerful detoxifier that helps to kick-start your metabolism. Along with hydrating your body, this drink will help to stimulate bowel movements. Drink one large glass, but if you feel like more, go for it— hydration is important.

- 12-ounce spring or filtered water, at room temperature
- Juice of 1 lemon
- 1/2-inch knob of ginger root

Add the lemon juice to the glass of water. Finely grate the ginger on a chopping board, then squeeze the ginger pieces in your hand, letting the juice of the ginger drip through your fingers and into the glass of water. Enjoy at room temperature upon rising for an amazing start to the day!

Nettle

Nettles are high in vitamins and minerals and have traditionally been used as a blood cleanser. Like other green foods, such as wheatgrass, they are a high-chlorophyll food. Chlorophyll builds blood, renews tissue, promotes healthy intestinal flora and improves liver function. These days nettles can be bought seasonally in farmers' markets or you can try foraging them for yourself.

Remember to wear gloves when picking and preparing your nettles to avoid their sting!

All you need for a nettle infusion tea is a handful of fresh or dried nettles. Put in a container and fill with boiling water. Cover and let steep for 10 minutes. Drink up to 3 cups a day for a nice spring detox.

DANDELION ROOT

Did you know that having allergies is a sign that the liver is compromised and has many toxins built up in it? Dandelion root stimulates bile production. The increased bile production helps clean the liver and flush out toxins. I recommend drinking dandelion root tea daily throughout this cleanse and using it once a week afterwards.

- 1 quart filtered water
- 2-3 teabags or 2-3 teaspoons loose dandelion root, dried
- 2 - 3 tablespoons honey

Bring water to a boil. Remove from heat and add tea bags. Cover and allow to steep until cool enough to drink, 20-30 minutes. Stir in honey and enjoy! I personally enjoy this tea at night to help my liver detox while I'm sleeping.

LICORICE ROOT

Licorice root has been used in both Eastern and Western medicine to treat a variety of illnesses ranging from the common cold to liver disease. Although Licorice has been used as a flavoring for hundreds of years, many people don't know that it also has very beneficial medicinal qualities and helps strengthen the body during times of stress. Licorice is also a powerful antiviral that contains 10 antioxidants, at least 25 fungicidal and 9 expectorant compounds.

- 1 cup chopped dry licorice root
- 1/2 cup cinnamon chips
- 1/2 cup dried orange peel
- 2 tablespoons whole cloves
- 1/2 cup chamomile flowers

Mix everything well in a bowl and store in a glass jar. To make the tea, combine 3 tablespoons of tea mix and 2 1/2 cups water in a pot. Bring to a boil over medium heat, reduce heat to low and allow to simmer for 10 minutes. Strain and pour into 2 cups and share with a friend.

Peppermint & Lemon Essential Oils

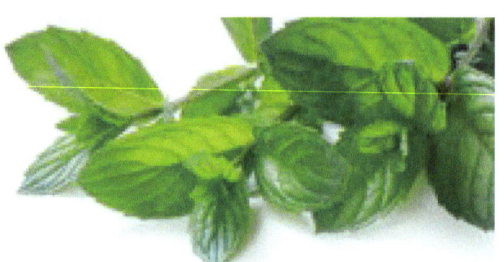

Peppermint oil releases drugs that are stored in your liver. Drugs that are stored in your liver block enzymes that are used to keep the liver functioning correctly. When the enzymes are blocked many people will experience weight gain or have allergies.

Lemon oil helps bile function from the liver to the gall bladder so it turns out bile salts that go into your intestines so that it can break down the proteins that you're going to eat that day. It helps **boost metabolism, reduces toxic build-up in fat cells, and aids liver function**.

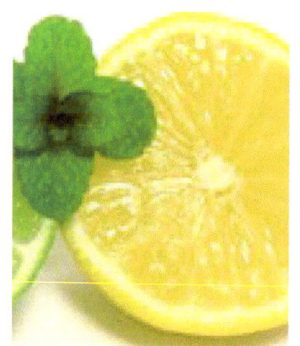

Add 1 drop peppermint and 2 drops lemon to 8 ounces of water. Repeat twice a day. (Make sure you find a really high quality source of essential oils as many on the market contain fillers and other chemicals. Email me for essential oil suggestions.)

(**Once again, the detox teas, herbs, and essentials oils are suggested, but not necessary to perform this cleanse.**)

COLON CLEANSING

A very important method in which the body removes waste and toxins from the body is through the colon. Having regular bowel movements is not necessarily an indication that your bowel is unobstructed and clear.

Since we are removing fiber from your diet during the SUPERhero 7 Day Cleanse, there will be nothing in your colon to stimulate the bowels. Therefore, to ensure that the toxins that are being released during the cleanse are removed from the body, you'll want to use one of the following methods.

There are many ways to clean out the colon. They include **colonics, enemas, laxative teas and salt water flushes,** to name a few. I'll describe the first three here but for sake of ease for this 7 day flush, **we will be using the laxative tea only**! If you are familiar and/or comfortable with colonics and enemas, that is a preferred method of colon cleansing over the tea.

COLONICS

This is a method of water irrigation of the colon that is done by a trained professional, called a Colon Hydrotherapist. To find certified colon hydrotherapists in your area go to the International Association for Colon Hydrotherapy website. (www.i-act.org)

ENEMAS

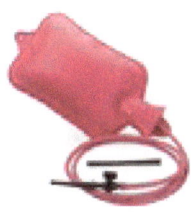

Enemas are another form of cleansing the colon using water or coffee. They are done easily at home with the use of an enema bag. A video is worth a thousand words, so watch the video here* to learn how easy it is to do yourself!

(*http://youtu.be/CDMa4wlQ7ts)

LAXATIVE TEA

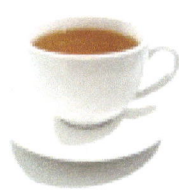

Laxative teas contain senna. Senna is a plant that stimulates the peristalsis action of the bowels. My favorite brands of **"poop tea"** are **Traditional Medicinals** and **Yogi Tea**. But any type of laxative tea will work. Drink a mug at night before bed.

AFFIRMATIONS

To get the most out of the cleanse, it's important that you are in a supportive environment and remain in a relaxed state.

The suggestions below will aid the body's natural detoxification processes and boost your mood and energy levels. You'll feel so good, you'll want to incorporate them into your new healthy lifestyle after you have completed the SUPERhero 7 day juice cleanse!

Your positive affirmation during this cleanse is:

**"I ACCEPT MYSELF UNCONDITIONALLY RIGHT NOW!
I AM A SUPERHERO!"**

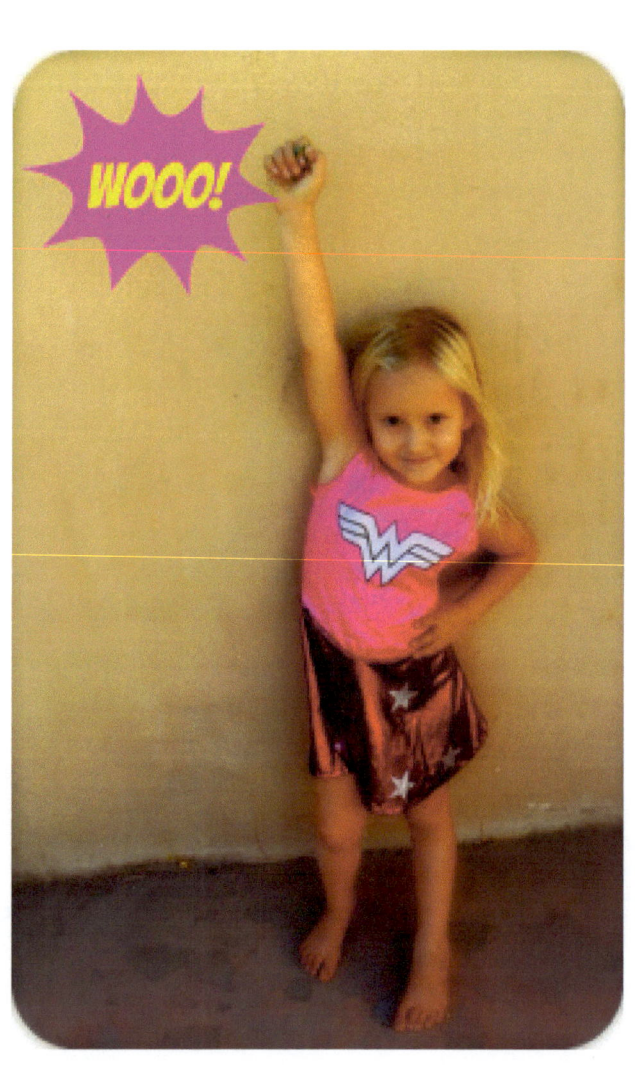

Say this out loud to yourself in the mirror when you wake up and before going to bed or whenever you find time throughout your day.

Also, just before you go to sleep, close your eyes and visualize your body as **radiantly healthy and clean and clear!**

If your goal is to lose weight, picture your body at your ideal weight. Hold this thought in your mind for 5 minutes.

Visualization is very important throughout this process as your subconscious mind responds to visual cues.

LET'S GET JUICING!

Enough of the idle chatter, right?

LET'S GET JUICING!

START SAVING THE PLANET (& YOUR HEALTH) ONE GREEN JUICE AT A TIME!!

Okay, okay, I get it. Here are your fabulous recipes. They are served best **cold and fresh, in your lucky rocket-ship underwear, and while sporting your favorite cape**.

Drink the juices throughout the day. **Drink** the same amount of **water**. On the days that call for a soup recipe. Make and **eat the soup**. If you're still hungry at any point, **make some more juice** using your creativity. You want to cleanse, not starve. We're all different sizes. If you don't finish your juice, that's okay, too. It's that simple.

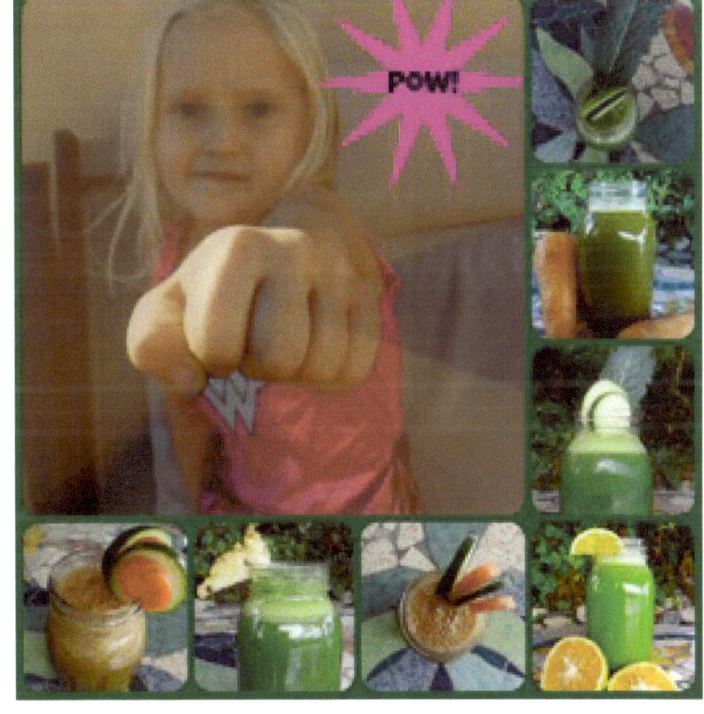

If you don't like a certain vegetable, have sensitivities to it, or cannot find it in your grocery store, **substitute it for something similar**.

One more thing – if a recipe calls for a fruit that is not in season (pineapple for example), feel free to use **frozen produce** (that you thawed the night before in the fridge), **canned produce** (not really recommended, however it's better than nothing), or **substitute it** for something else in season (like apples or grapes).

You really can't go wrong if you have a GREEN JUICE in hand!

Day 1

The Kancer Ka-Pow!

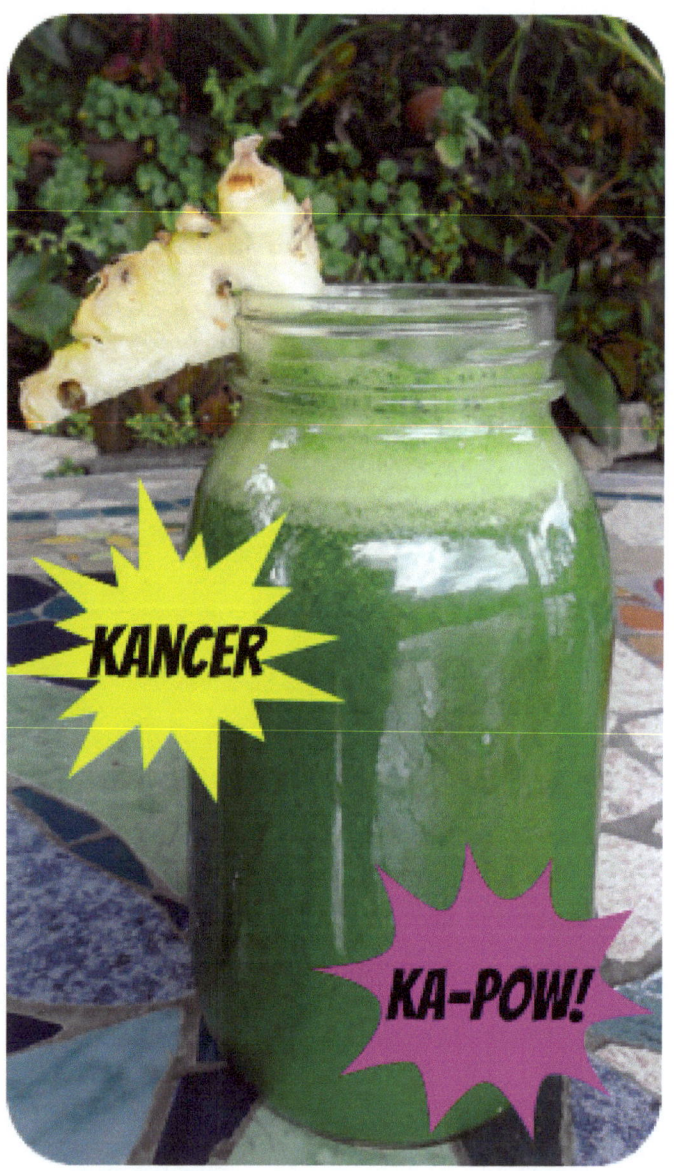

The SuperStars

- 2 **large apples**
- 1 **pineapple**
- 8 cups **chopped kale**
- 4 **limes**
- 20 **basil leaves** (a small handful)
- 2 cups **water**

Run all items through the juicer. Add 2 cups water to the juice. Makes 48 ounces of juice. Drink this throughout the day. Finish by dinner time.

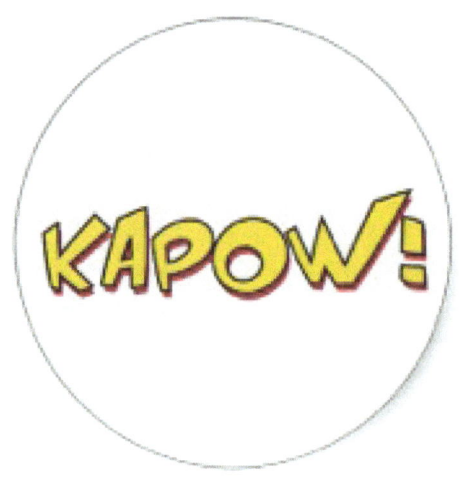

22

THE SEE-THROUGH-WALLS FACTOR

- Apples are full of **antioxidants** – disease–fighting compounds that prevent and repair oxidation damage that happens during normal cell activity
- Apples **kick both diarrhea and constipation in the butt**!
- Apples help the **liver detoxify toxins**.
- Pineapple juice has an anthelmintic effect – meaning it helps **get rid of intestinal worms**. Yuck! And Woooooo–hooooooo!
- Pineapple is loaded with manganese, a mineral critical in the **development of strong bones and connective tissue**. Important for all superheroes.
- Pineapple contains a proteolytic enzyme bromelain which is **anti–inflammatory**. This comes in handy when your body is sore from fighting crime all night long.
- Kale is high in **iron**. Iron is essential for good health and transporting oxygen to various parts of your body.
- Kale is fantastically full of Vitamin K. You know what the K stands for?? **Cancer–Killer**! Vitamin K helps to protect the body against various cancers.
- Not only are limes known for fighting scurvy, they are also **anti–carcinogenic**. Just like my friend Kale, mentioned above.
- Lime juice also is an **enemy of kidney stones**. Fresh lime juice contains more citric acid than orange or grapefruit juice. Citric acid is a natural inhibitor of kidney stones, which are made of crystallized calcium.
- Basil **protects against unwanted bacterial growth** in your body in addition to inhibiting several species of pathogenic bacteria that have become resistant to commonly used antibiotic drugs.
- Basil is also loaded with you know what? **Vitamin K, the cancer killer**!!

Dinner – Time

The Sweet Potato Sunset!

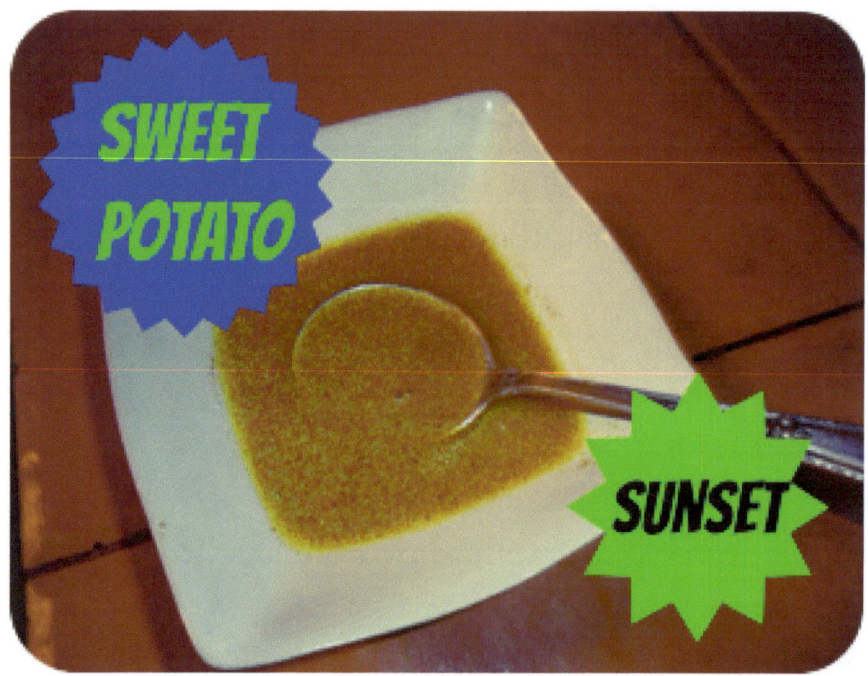

The SuperStars

- 1 **sweet potato**
- 1 **apple**
- 1 **carrot**
- 1 **green pepper**
- 3 **cloves garlic**
- 1 **onion**
- 1 teaspoon **cumin**
- 1 teaspoon **turmeric**
- 2 tablespoons **coconut oil**
- **salt and pepper** to taste
- **nutritional yeast** to garnish

Run all items (sweet potato through onion) through the juicer. Pour into pan and heat slightly on stovetop. Stir in cumin, turmeric, coconut oil, salt and pepper to taste. Sprinkle with nutritional yeast. Makes enough for 1 SUPERhero.

The See-Through-Walls Factor

- Sweet potatoes are loaded, and I mean jam-packed, with **Vitamin A**. This one little sweet potato you are using up there…contains over 400% of what you need for a day of Vitamin A. It's called Vitamin A (first on the list) for a reason. Vitamin A keeps our skin, mucous membranes, and immune system strong. Without a healthy supply of Vitamin A in our diet, nasty bacteria and viruses would take over!

- Sweet potatoes **regulate blood sugar**. (Helpful while juice cleansing as the fiber is removed from the juices, which can lead to blood-sugar spikes.)

- Sweet potatoes are also full of **antioxidants,** helping us to fight disease, look younger, feel younger and leap over buildings in a single bound!

- Apples are packed with **Vitamin C, and Vitamin A, and flavonoids** and with smaller amounts of **phosphorus, iron and calcium**.

- For centuries, onions have been used to **reduce inflammation and heal infections**.

- Raw onion encourages the production of **good cholesterol** (**HDL**), thus keeping your heart healthy.

- Garlic **strengthens the immune system** as well as helps to fight chest infections, coughs and congestion. An old folk remedy is to **eat a clove of garlic dipped in honey at the first sign of a cold or flu**.

- **Turmeric** is 5 to 8 times stronger than Vitamin E and stronger than Vitamin C in regards to **boosting your immune system! Can we say "Ka-Pow!!"**

- **Turmeric** also supports healthy joint function, promotes radiant skin (that looks great in a mask) and helps improve digestion.

- **The antiseptic properties of cumin** can help fight flu, by boosting your immune system.

- Cumin helps with **digestive disorders** – helps control stomach pain, indigestion, diarrhea, nausea, and morning sickness.

- **Nutritional Yeast is a vegetarian source of B-12**. That's right. No animals need to be harmed in the acquisition of your Vitamin B. The cows thank you.

Day 2

The Orange Giant!

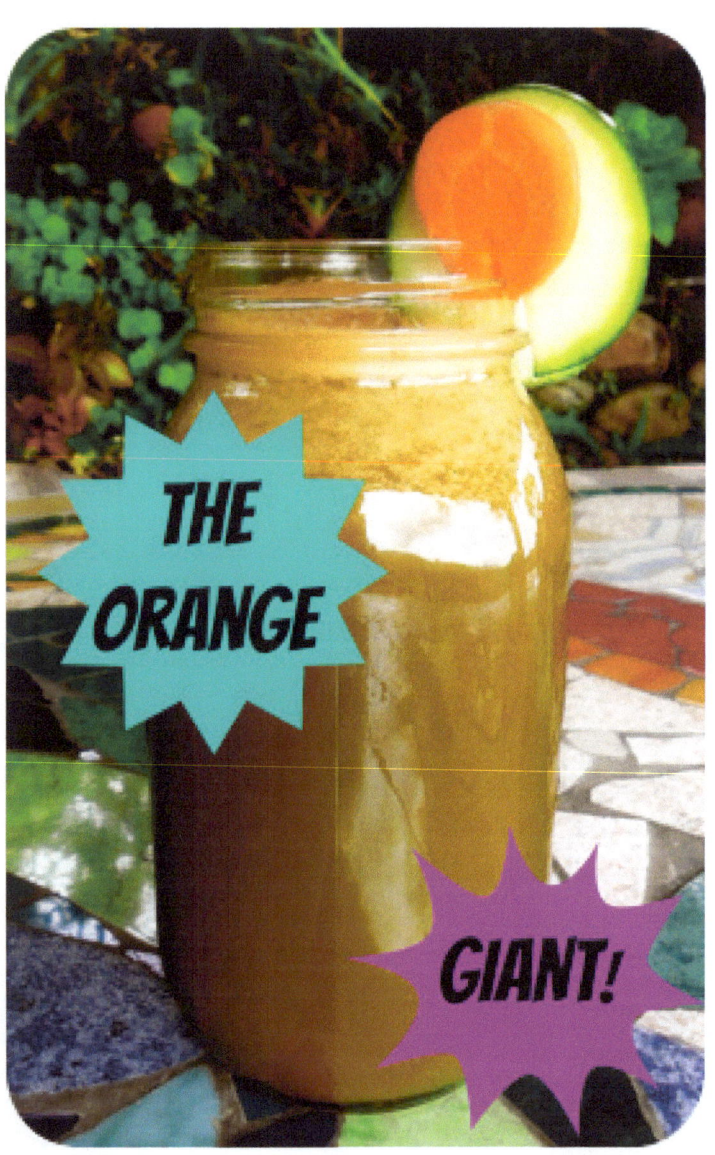

The SuperStars

- 2–3 heads of **lettuce** (depending on size)
- 2 large **cucumbers**
- 8 large **carrots**
- 8 stalks **celery**
- 1 **lime**

Run all items through the juicer and drink throughout the day until the sun goes down. Makes approximately 8 cups of juice.

At night, drink a couple cups of your preferred detox tea – nettle, dandelion root, etc.

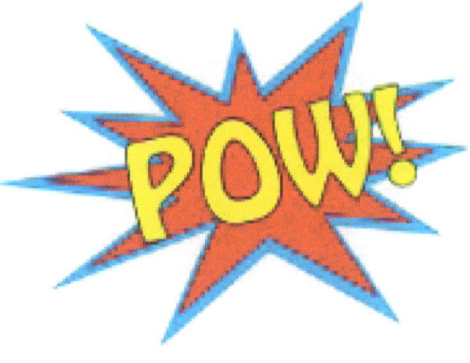

THE SEE-THROUGH-WALLS FACTOR

- Think lettuce is lowly? Think again. Lettuce leaves are the store house of many **phyto-nutrients** that have health promoting and disease prevention properties.
- Vitamins in lettuce are plentiful. Fresh leaves are an excellent source of **Vitamin A, beta-carotenes, Vitamin K, folates and Vitamin C.**
- Carrots also rock the **beta-carotene,** helping to keep the eyes and skin healthy.
- Carrots also **balance the acid / alkaline ratio in the body**. We need a body that is slightly alkaline. Many of our diets are way to acid. Carrots to the rescue!
- Cucumbers have **most of the vitamins the body needs in a single day**. Add them to all of your juices. Really.
- Cucumbers are a **great source of B vitamins** meaning they are an energetic boost when you need it!
- Celery is another **anti-inflammatory delight**. Kiss muscle pain good-bye by adding celery into your vegetable juices!
- Not only for margaritas, limes have an irresistible scent which causes your mouth to water and this actually aids primary digestion. The natural acidity in lime does the rest. The flavonoids in limes, the compounds found in the fragrant oils extracted from lime, stimulate the digestive system and increase secretion of digestive juices, bile and acids. This flood of flavonoids also **stimulate the peristaltic motion of the bowels** helping to get the toxins out!

Day 3

The Wam-Bam!

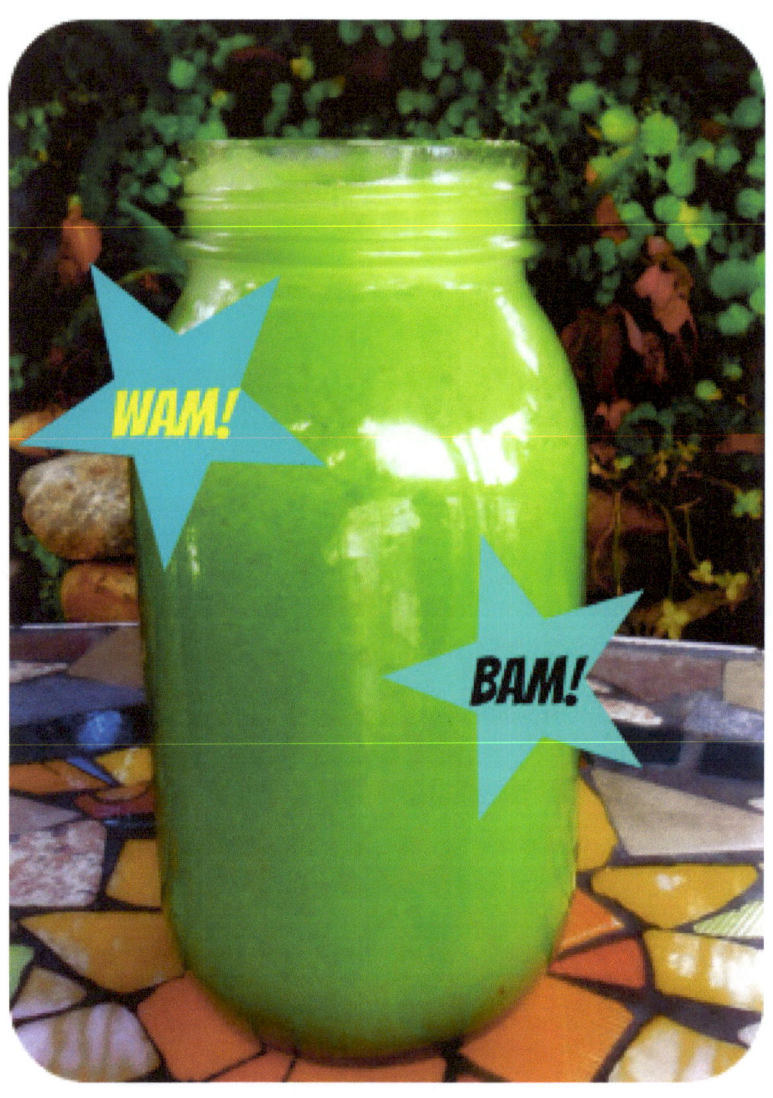

The SuperStars

- 1 large **pineapple**
- 4 **limes**
- 3 cups packed **spinach**
- 8 stalks **celery**

Makes 6 cups of pure blissful green nectar from the sun.

Enjoy throughout the day. But save room for dinner!

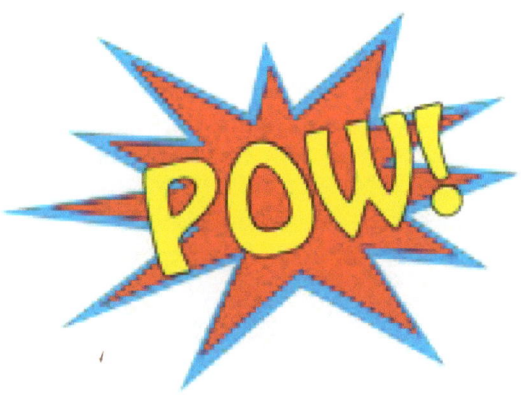

THE SEE-THROUGH-WALLS FACTOR

- You will easily get **more than 100% of your daily requirements for Vitamin C** with this amount of pineapple. Vitamin C is your body's primary water-soluble antioxidant, fighting crime, and free radicals that attack and damage normal cells. Makes you wanna say: **WAM**!

- Pineapple has also been rumored (ok, proven) to **protect your eyes**. Yup, studies show that pineapples protect against macular degeneration.

- The ample amount of acids present in lime helps **clear the excretory system** by washing and cleaning off the tracts, just as some acids are used to clean floors and toilets. Think of limes as a scrub brush for your intestines.

- Pop-Eye was right. Eating copious amounts of spinach is good for you! Rich in vitamins and minerals, it is also concentrated in health-promoting phytonutrients such as carotenoids (beta-carotene, lutein, and zeaxanthin) and flavonoids to provide you with **powerful antioxidant protection**.

- **Bright, vibrant-looking spinach leaves are not only more appealing to the eye but more nourishing as well**. Recent research has shown that spinach leaves that look fully alive and vital have greater concentrations of Vitamin C than spinach leaves that are pale in color. Make sure you opt for the dark green leaves when choosing your spinach.

- Celery has **blood pressure reducing properties**. It contains active phthalides, which relax the muscles of the arteries that regulate blood pressure so the vessels dilate. Phthalides also reduce stress hormones, which can cause blood vessels to constrict. You know what else reduces blood pressure? **Sitting outside, reading a book while drinking your green juice**. BAM!!

DINNER - TIME

THE CREAMY CARROT SHA-ZAM!

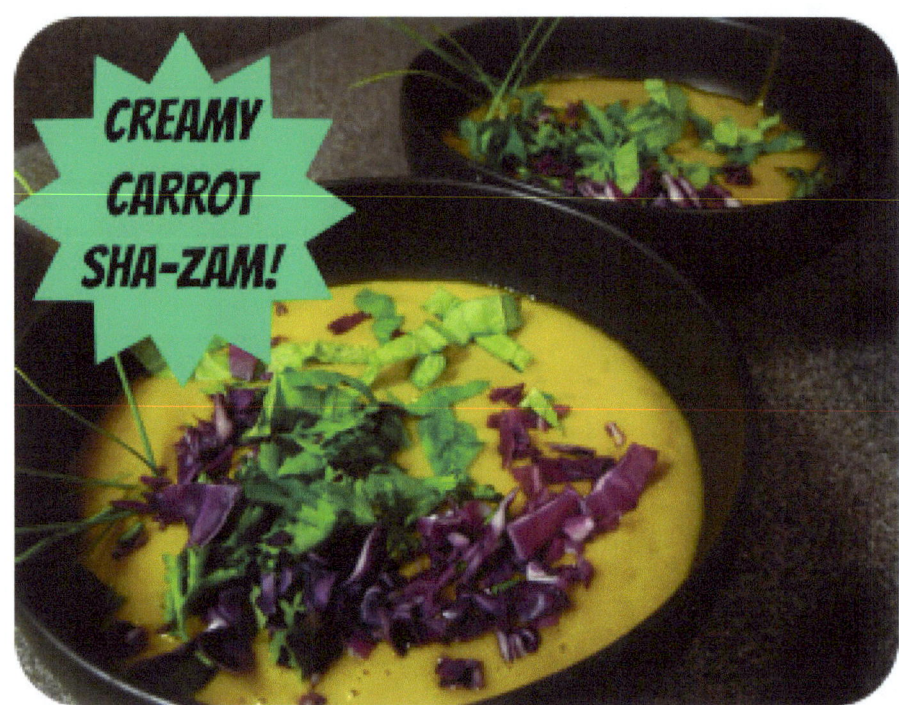

THE SUPERSTARS

Juice:

- 7 to 8 **carrots** (about 1/2 pound)
- 1/2 large **cucumber**
- 1/2 inch **ginger**
- 2 cloves **garlic**
- 1/2 **lemon**

Blend With:

- 1 small **avocado**
- 1 tablespoon **coconut oil**
- 1/2 teaspoon **cumin**
- 1/2 teaspoon **sea salt**
- 1/2 teaspoon **black pepper**
- a dash **cayenne**

Taste and adjust the spices accordingly. The picture shows the soup garnished with cilantro, chives, basil and purple cabbage. Looks pretty, huh? Sorry to tease you, but save those for next week. In this cleanse, we'll keep our fiber intake only to the avocado.

THE SEE-THROUGH-WALLS FACTOR

- **A carrot a day**.....**helps you see through walls!** Loaded with Vitamin A, which help to keep your eyes healthy!

- Cucumbers not only make a nice 'pop' when you snap them in half, they also help to **rehydrate the body and replenish daily vitamins**.

- **Cucumbers fight bad breath!** The phytochemicals in cukes kill the bacteria in your mouth responsible for bad breath. When paired with garlic, they should counter-act each other nicely.

- Ginger **improves the absorption and assimilation of essential nutrients** in the body.

- Got a bad case of gas? (All this cleansing can certainly do that as harmful bacteria is swept out of the gut.) Luckily for you, **ginger helps reduce flatulence**.

- Popular folklore says that **garlic is good for more than scaring hungry vampires away! Impotency has long been thought to benefit from doses of garlic, and treatment continues in many communities to this day**. Why not try treating yourself with garlic for several months before you head off to the doctor for that Viagra prescription?

- **Cardiovascular disease can be reduced by ingesting garlic**. LDL cholesterol is no friend of garlic and the aortic plaque deposits that gather on the walls of your body's veins can be reduced with the use of garlic too. Studies have shown the amazing benefits of taking garlic in relation to heart disease.

- Some call the avocado the alphabet fruit because of all the vitamins it contains. **One avocado provides your body with Vitamins A, C, E, K and B6, along with an enormous amount of potassium and "healthy" fat.**

- Perhaps the biggest health benefit of avocados is that by **adding avocado to certain foods, you can improve your absorption of nutrients**.

- **Avocados provide all 18 essential amino acids** necessary for the body to form a complete protein.

- Cayenne fights **inflammation and is a natural pain reliever** (remember that next time you go to pop an aspirin).

- The lauric acid in coconut oil can **kill bacteria, viruses and fungi,** helping to fight off infections!

Day 4

Pineapple Brilliance!

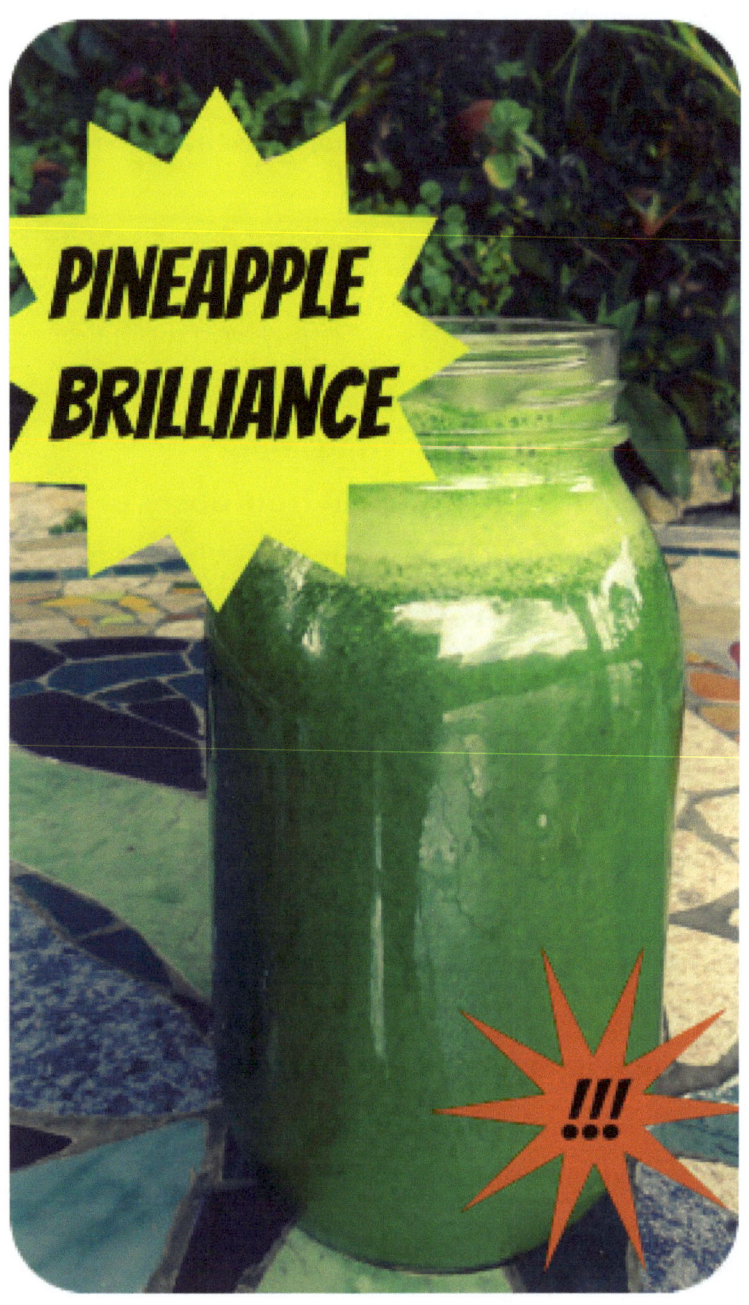

The SuperStars

.1 medium **pineapple**
.1 bunch **swiss chard**
.2 large **cucumbers**
.2 large **apples**

Juice 'em up and drink it down! Take your time. Enjoy. Savor this sweet delight....as this is all you are going to be drinking today.

Remember to drink your water. Make a couple of glasses of detox tea for the night followed by a laxative tea before bed.

And once again – if you ever get too hungry, simply make yourself some more juice!

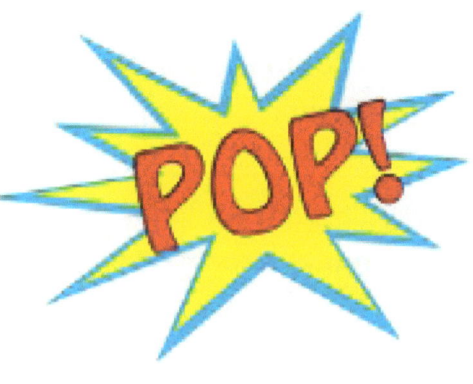

THE SEE-THROUGH-WALLS FACTOR

- I know, I know, pineapple again!? Yes!! Because pineapple is amazing! It's a SUPER fruit and I love it. **Pineapple is high in manganese,** a mineral that is critical to development of strong bones and connective tissue. A cup of fresh pineapple will give you nearly 75% of the recommended daily amount.

- Pineapple is said to **discourage blood clot development**. This makes it a valuable player for frequent fliers and others at risk for blood clots.

- **Fresh pineapple juice has been traditionally used for morning sickness**.

- If you have a cold with a productive cough, add pineapple to your diet. Fresh pineapple is not only high in Vitamin C, but the bromelain in pineapple has the ability to **reduce mucus in the throat.**

- Swiss chard contains a unique source of phytonutrients called betalains. Many of the betalain pigments in chard have been shown to provide antioxidant, anti-inflammatory, and detoxification support.

- Swiss chard is not only one of the most popular vegetables along the Mediterranean but it is **one of the most nutritious vegetables around** and ranks second only to spinach following the analysis of the total nutrient-richness of the World's healthiest vegetables (or so states the World's Healthiest Foods website).

- The amount of Vitamin K in a cup of swiss chard is scary. I wouldn't be surprised if after eating just a fork-full of swiss chard, that you'd **start growing new bones** that you never had before! (Vitamin K is important in bone health and non-collagen protein creation.)

- **Cucumbers help to cure diabetes, reduce cholesterol and control blood pressure!** Cucumber juice contains a hormone which is needed by the cells of the pancreas for producing insulin which has been found to be beneficial to diabetic patients. Researchers found that a compound called sterols in cucumbers may help reduce cholesterol levels. Cucumbers contain a lot of potassium, magnesium and fiber. These work effectively for regulating blood pressure. This makes cucumbers good for treating both low blood pressure and high blood pressure. **Brilliant!**

DAY 5

THE INCREDIBLE EDIBLE INFLAMMATION ASSASSIN!

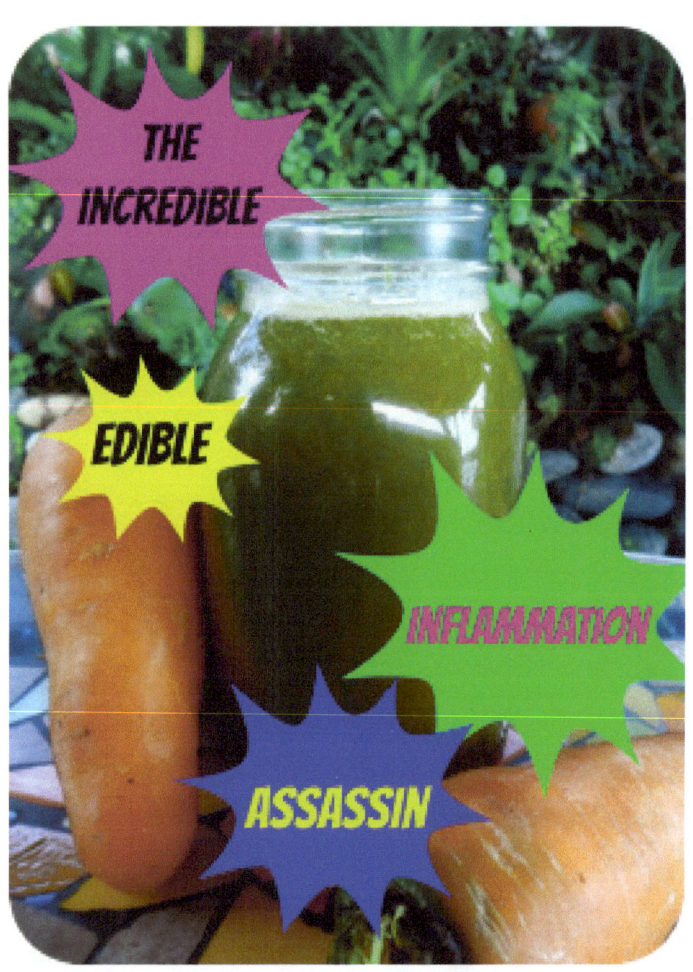

THE SUPERSTARS

- 2 large **yellow** or **green peppers**
- 3 large **cucumbers**
- 16 large **carrots**
- 2 large **apples**
- 1 **lemon**
- 1/2 inch **ginger**
- handful **cilantro**
- 4 ounces **water**

Makes 64 ounces of vegetable juice. Once again, this will be your sole form of sustenance for the day.

Don't worry, you'll have a delicious soup tomorrow night. Make sure and drink some warm detox tea at night. If you're really really really really really craving some sweetness, add a teaspoon of honey to the tea.

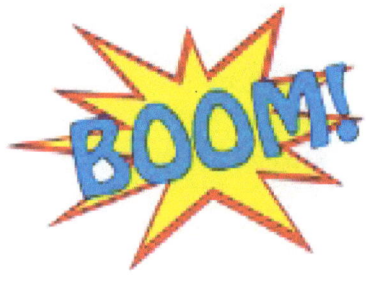

THE SEE-THROUGH-WALLS FACTOR

- Cucumbers **promote joint health and relieve gout and arthritis pain**. Cucumbers are an excellent source of silica, which are known to help promote joint health by strengthening the connective tissues. They are also rich in vitamin A, B1, B6, C & D, folate, calcium, magnesium, and potassium. **When mixed with carrot juice, they can relieve gout and arthritis pain by lowering the uric acid levels**.

- Speaking of joint health, are you reeling under joint pain? **Ginger, with its anti-inflammatory properties—can bring relief**. Try floating some ginger into your bath to help aching muscles and joints. Or better yet, drink it down in your juice!

- Carrots and other orange-hued vegetables are rich in Vitamin A and beta-carotene, both of which are believed to **fight inflammation** (are you catching onto the pattern here?).

- Sweet peppers are also known as capsicum, bell pepper, red pepper, cayenne, hot pepper, and green pepper. In addition, it's also known for its nutritional benefits. Red peppers contain the highest amount of Vitamin C, followed by yellow and then green. Sweet peppers also have a high beta carotene content…which translates to PAIN RELIEF! Studies have shown that eating sweet peppers can help with arthritis. **The capsiate that sweet peppers contain is anti-inflammatory in nature and helps for both pain relief and relief from inflammation**.

- Can you guess what cilantro can be used for?? **Its anti-inflammatory effects!** Studies show that cilantro helps with the inflammation caused by arthritis. **Boom!**

DAY 6

THE GREEN MARVEL!

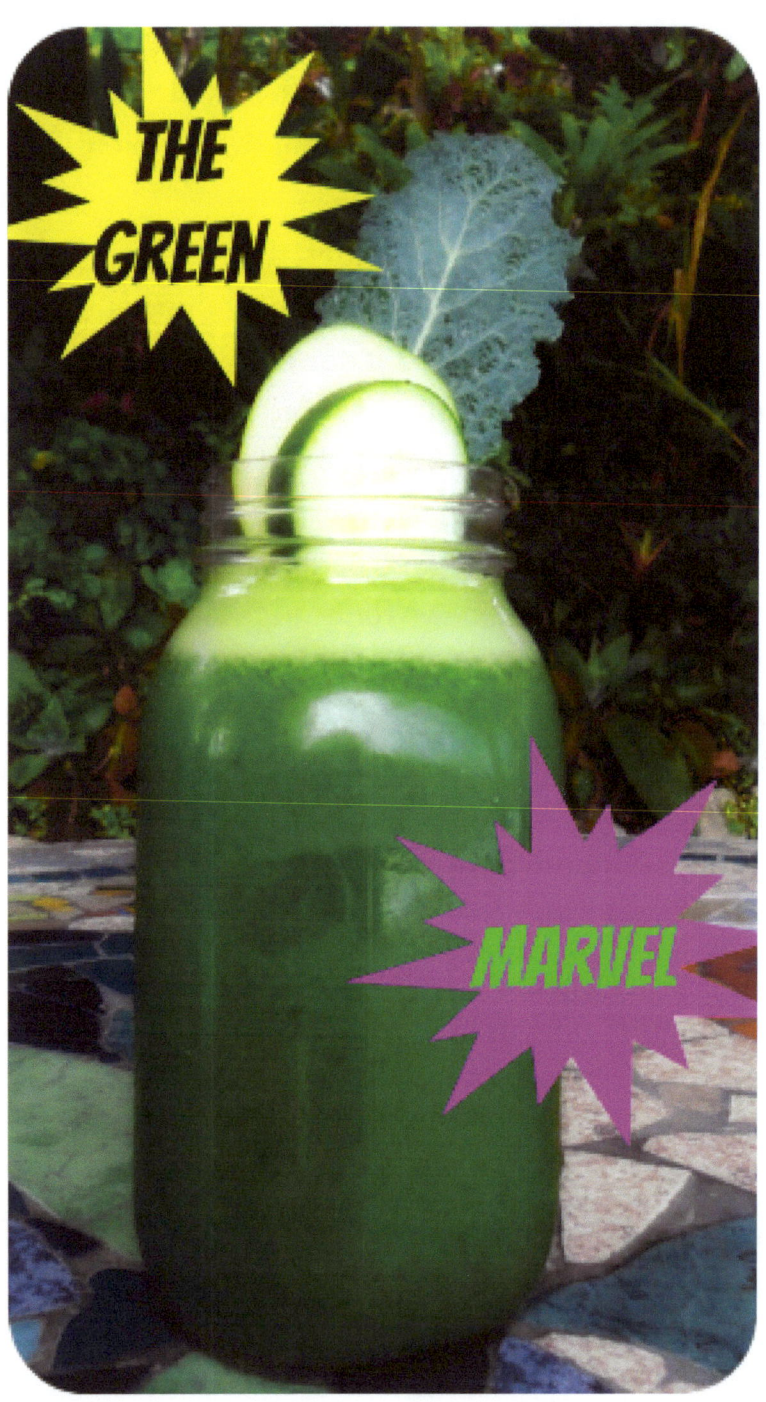

THE SUPERSTARS

- 8 small **apples**
- 6 cups chopped **kale**
- 1 large **cucumber**
- 4 **limes**
- 1/4 – 1/2 inch **ginger**
- 4 ounces **water**

Makes 40 ounces total of this marvelous green delight!

Sip and enjoy throughout the day but save room for dinner!

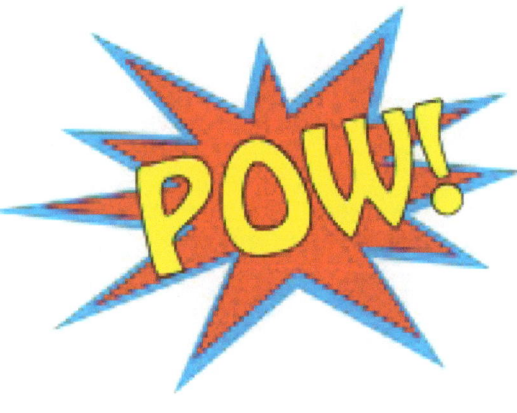

THE SEE-THROUGH-WALLS FACTOR

- **Kale has more iron than beef**. Think about that the next time you are flexing your biceps as you sit down to steak and potatoes.
- **Kale is filled with powerful antioxidants**. These help protect against various cancers. (If kale had arms, he would be flexing and showing his strength at this moment.)
- **Kale has more calcium than milk**. Calorie for calorie, it kicks milks butt in calcium amounts.
- **Kale is high in Vitamin A and Vitamin C**.
- **Kale will solve all your financial problems**!! (Ok, I made that one up.)
- **Apples help you to breathe easier**. Really! Apples contain an antioxidant called quercetin, which aids endurance by making oxygen more available to the lungs.
- **Cucumbers prevent hangovers**! You think it strange to say? To avoid a morning hangover or headache; eat a few cucumber slices before going to bed. Cucumbers contain enough sugar, B vitamins and electrolytes to replenish many essential nutrients, reducing the intensity of both hangover and headache.
- There are two main causes of gout. The first source is the accumulation of free radicals in the body, and the second is the accumulation of toxins in the body, primarily uric acid. **Limes can help prevent both of these causes**!
- **Ginger helps with a variety of tummy issues** including: cramps, indigestion, hangovers, airsickness and nausea in general.
- **Got a fever? Reach for a couple limes**! Citrus fruits in general have fever-reducing qualities, and if the fever is very high, your diet should be restricted to lemon juice and water. **Pretty marvelous, huh?**

Dinner - Time

The Terrific Tomato Soup!

The SuperStars

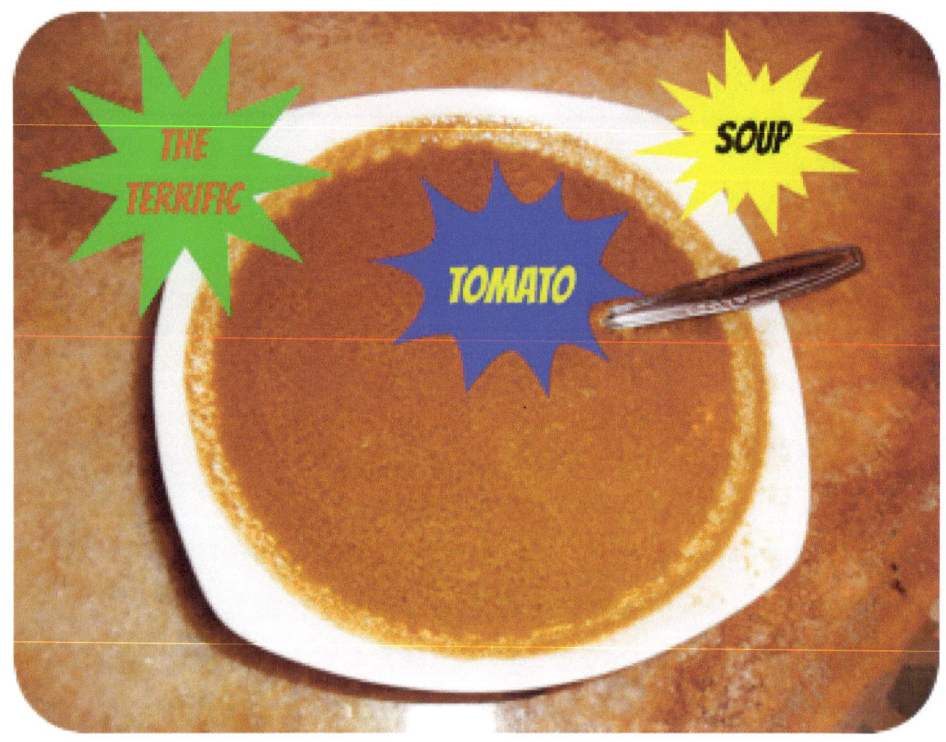

Juice:
- 1 **tomato**
- 1 **carrot**
- 2 **green peppers**
- 3 cloves **garlic**
- 1/2 small **onion**

Stir in:
- 1/2 cup **water**
- 1 tablespoon **coconut oil**
- **salt and pepper** to taste
- dash **cayenne**
- 1 or 2 tablespoons **nutritional yeast**

Heat slightly on the stove. Makes enough for approximately 1 superhero. Enjoy it baby, enjoy!

THE SEE-THROUGH-WALLS FACTOR

- Want your skin to look amazing behind that superhero mask!? **Tomatoes make your skin look great**. Beta_carotene, also found in carrots and sweet potatoes, helps protect skin against sun damage. Tomatoes' lycopene also makes skin less sensitive to UV light damage, a leading cause of fine lines and wrinkles.

- Tomatoes **build strong bones**. Vitamin K and calcium in tomatoes are both very good for strengthening and repairing bones.

- **Fungal and bacterial vaginal infections don't stand a chance** when treated with garlic! When crushed or bruised, garlic releases **allicin** which is a sulphuric compound that is a natural antibiotic.

- **Garlic regulates blood sugar** as it enhances the level of insulin in the blood. This may assist in the control of diabetes.

- **Garlic is a great source of Vitamin B6** which is needed for a healthy immune system and the efficient growth of new cells. Vitamin B6 can also assist with mood swings and improve your cheery disposition!

- Nutritional Yeast is a **great source of folic acid**. This is important in cell maintenance and production.

- **Populations that eat a LOT of coconut are among the healthiest people on the planet**. The Tokelauans, who live in the South Pacific, are in excellent health with no evidence of heart disease. Considering heart disease is the number one killer in the United States, I think we have a couple things to learn about healthy saturated fats and their role in heart health.

- **Coconut oil can help you burn fat!** The medium_chain triglycerides (MCTs) in coconut oil can increase energy expenditure compared to the same amount of calories from longer chain fats. **Wouldn't you say that's terrific?!**

- Cayenne has become a **popular home treatment for mild high blood pressure and high blood cholesterol levels**. Cayenne preparations prevent platelets from clumping together and accumulating in the blood, allowing the blood to flow more easily. Since it is thought to help improve circulation, its often used by those who have cold hands and feet.

DAY 7

THE SMOOTH MOVE!

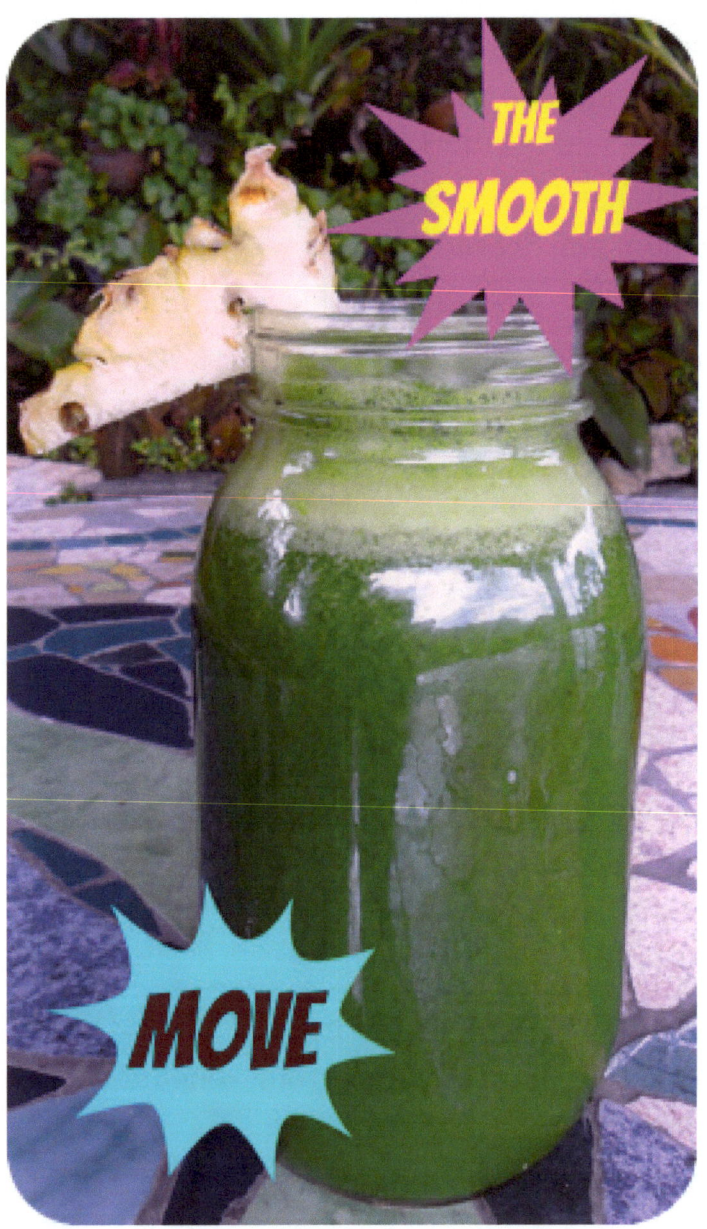

THE SUPERSTARS

- 8 green **apples**
- 6 cups packed **spinach**
- 8 stalks **celery**
- 1 handful **parsley**
- 1 handful **basil**
- 2 **lemons**

Makes 8 cups of amazing juice. Sip on it throughout the day. When the sun goes down, drink a couple cups of detox tea and bathe in the realization that you are done and that you did it!

Seven days wasn't so bad, now was it?

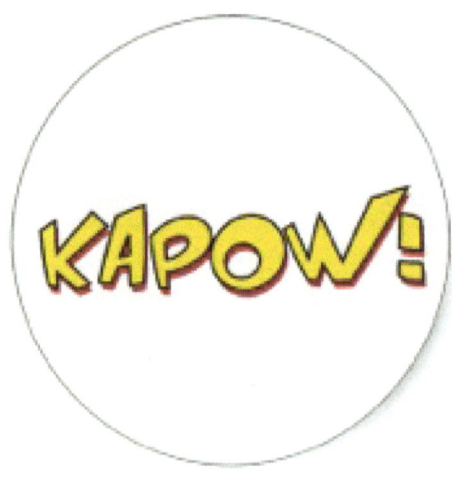

40

THE SEE-THROUGH-WALLS FACTOR

- **Apples prevent heart attacks!!** Last year, the Iowa Womens Health Study reported that among the 34,000 women it has been tracking for nearly 20 years, apples were associated with a lower risk of death from both coronary heart disease and cardiovascular disease. Brilliant!!

- A lesser known fact about spinach – **Spinach eases constipation and protects the mucus lining of the stomach, so that you stay free of ulcers.** It also flushes toxins out from the colon.

- Another lesser known benefit of spinach is its role in skin care. **The bounty of vitamins and minerals in spinach can bring you quick relief from dry, itchy skin and lavish you with a radiant complexion.**

- **Celery is incredibly alkalizing to the body,** helping to balance the body's pH.

- Celery is rich in sodium, which is very different than table salt. Normal table salt is composed of insoluble inorganic compounds which lead to the development of varicose veins, hardening of the arteries and other aliments. On the other hand, the sodium that is available in celery is soluble and organic (live), and is essential for the body. **Organic salt allows the body to use the other nutrients that are taken into the body.** Every cell in our body is constantly bathed in a salt solution, and if the salt level is not in balance, dehydration occurs. This is why celery juice is a perfect rehydration drink!

- Parsley **supports the kidneys** by helping to flush toxins out of the body.

- **Basil protects your DNA.** Bet you didn't know that one. The unique array of active flavonoids, including orientin and vicenin, have been shown to protect cell structures and cell chromosomes from radiation and oxygen-based damage.

- Looking to lose weight? The citric acid present in lemons is an **excellent fat burner.** You can consume two glasses a day and see legitimate and remarkable results within a week.

- The high potassium content of lemons are very effective in **removal of the toxic substances and the precipitates which get deposited in kidneys and the urinary bladder.** Know what that means? Lower occurrence of UTIs, kidney stones and prostate issues. **Pretty smooooooth, huh?**

THE CHEAT-SHEET RECAP FOR THE WEEK

We just went over a lot in these previous 40 pages or so. I know this. That's why I've created this 'cheat-sheet' for you for the 7 days. You can refer to the sheet here, and you can also go to my website to print one out and post it on your fridge! (That way you don't have to make this nice and clean book all dirty.)

The PureRadiantSelf SUPERhero 7 Day Juice Cleanse

The SUPER To-Do List	Day 1	Day 2	Day 3	Day 4	Day 5	Day 6	Day 7
Morning Affirmation	☐	☐	☐	☐	☐	☐	☐
Daily Green Juice	☐	☐	☐	☐	☐	☐	☐
30 Minutes Exercise	☐	☐	☐	☐	☐	☐	☐
30 Minutes Yoga	☐	☐	☐	☐	☐	☐	☐
Nightly Soup (Days 1, 3, and 6)	☐	☐	☐	☐	☐	☐	☐
Laxative Tea (nightly)	☐	☐	☐	☐	☐	☐	☐
Nightly Affirmation	☐	☐	☐	☐	☐	☐	☐
Detox Tea (As desired)	☐	☐	☐	☐	☐	☐	☐

To print out your own cheat-sheet, soar your way over to this webpage here:
www.pureradiantself.com/juicing/7dayjuicecleanse/

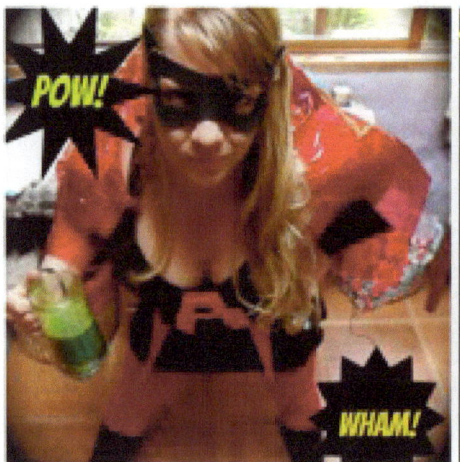
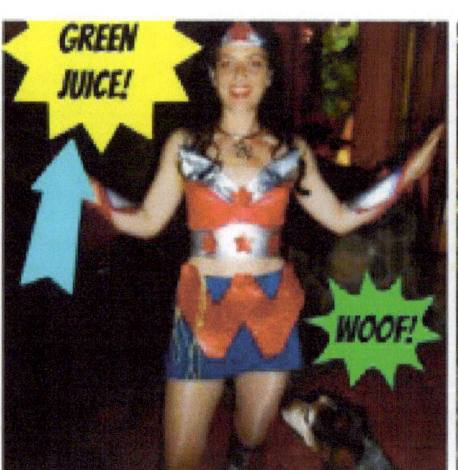
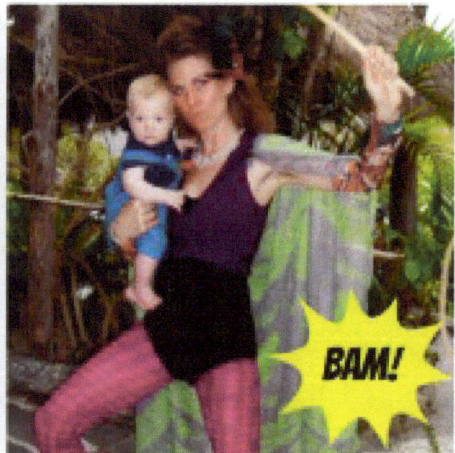

THE SHOPPING LIST

Food Items	Quantity	Additional Items	Quantity
Apple	23	Cayenne Pepper	To Taste
Avocado	1	Cumin	To Taste
Basil	2 handfuls	Salt and Pepper	To Taste
Carrot	42 large	Turmeric	To Taste
Celery	24 stalks	Coconut Oil	3 Tablespoons
Cilantro	1 handful	Nutritional Yeast	3 Tablespoons
Cucumber	8 1/2	Laxative Tea	7 Tea bags
Garlic	8 cloves	**Detox Tea(s)**	**Quantity**
Ginger	1 1/2 inch	Dandelion Root	As Desired
Green Pepper	5	Ginger/Lemon Tea	As Desired
Kale	14 cups	Licorice Root Tea:	As Desired
Lemon	4	- Cinnamon chips	1/2 cup
Lettuce	2 or 3 heads	- Dried Orange Peel	1/2 cup
Lime	13	- Cloves	2 tablespoons
Onion	1 1/2	- Chamomile Flowers	1/2 cup
Parsley	1 handful	- Dry Licorice Root	1 cup
Pineapple	3	Nettle	As Desired
Spinach	9 cups	Honey	As Desired
Sweet Potato	1	Peppermint Essential Oil (EO)	8 drops a day
Swiss Chard	1 bunch	Lemon EO	8 drops a day
Tomato	1		

BREAKING THE FAST

Yes. YES. **YES**!!! **You did it**! You've successfully completed the 7 Day Superhero Juice Cleanse! And I wish I could tell you that your work here is done. However, I cannot say that. And I won't. Uh_uh. Nope. But good thing you're a superhero because it'll now take some superhero will power to **SAFELY** and **GRACEFULLY** and **CORRECTLY** ease into eating food again.

"YOU MEAN I CAN'T JUST GO BACK TO EATING STEAK AND POTATOES?"

Nope, I'm afraid not. But don't get your cape in a bunch. Let me share with you how to ease your belly back into digesting food (aka fiber).

DAYS 1 & 2 – **Eat only raw foods**. Continue to drink juices but add fiber into your diet in the form of smoothies and salads. Imagine that you are still juicing. Stay in the mind_frame of 'liquids' mainly. Don't get excited about going out to a fancy dinner consisting of a five course meal. That is still days away. Your stomach will revolt. Strongly. And you will not like the results.

DAYS 3 & 4 – **Same as above**. However, now you can **add in some cooked vegetables and grains**. (You should be saying '**Woooo weeeeee, holy cooked food, Batman**!' at this point.) I suggest veggie and quinoa soup, baked sweet potatoes or steamed rice and vegetables.

DAYS 5 & 6 – **Start to branch out to more 'exotic' cuisine** but don't get too crazy. Still avoid meat, eggs, dairy, caffeine, and alcohol like your arch nemesis. So what does this mean? Well, it simply means more elaborate vegetarian cuisine beyond the 'simple' and 'basics.'

DAYS 7 AND BEYOND – "Mother may I PLEASE PLEASE PLEASE start to eat my fish, bread, yogurt, and everything else I'm craving?" Why, yes, now you may if you promise to eat slowly and with consciousness." Really, go slow. Start to incorporate your 'normal' foods back into your diet. Whatever 'normal' means to you. Be aware of how your body responds to the standard allergens (gluten, dairy, nuts, alcohol) in addition to how you feel after eating foods that contain sugar and caffeine. You may be surprised at the foods your body doesn't like anymore.

MY AMAZING EXPERIENCE

I can't lie. It would be against my SUPERhero morals. I love this cleanse. I love it. I love it! I. LOVE. IT! After those short seven days: I have more energy, my skin clears up, I feel great, I have more control of my emotions and honestly....

I FEEL LIKE A SUPERhero!

I love this cleanse compared to other cleanses because I still get to 'eat' during it. I don't feel like I'm starving myself. I still go about my daily life without much interruption. And let me tell you, after successfully completing a 40 Day Juice Cleanse, this felt like nothing. Nothing I tell ya, nothing. Bring on the evil mad‑man with the crazy plan to destroy the planet! Show me the meteor threatening to crash into us and blow us to smithereens! I'm ready.

SUPERHERO POWERS ACTIVATED!

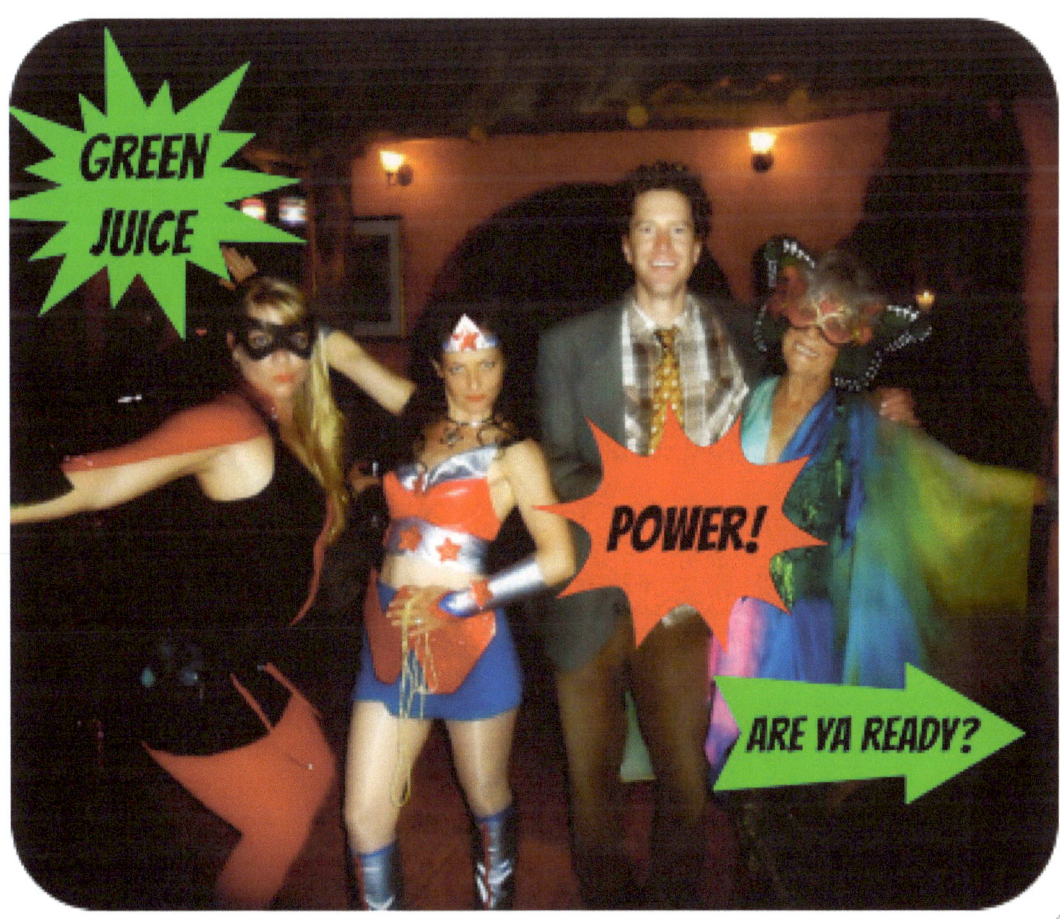

*Peter Parker hanging out with his favorite
Super Heroines*

Where To Go From Here?

You start! If you don't already have a juicer, buy yourself a juicer. Look at the calendar and pick a start date. Circle it with a permanent marker. Maybe put a couple stars or hearts around that date. Why? Because not only will that date be the start towards elevating you to **SUPERhero status**…but it will also be the date you have agreed to loving yourself just a little bit more by giving yourself the gift of health.

Tell your friends and family members about your SUPERhero 7-Day Juice Cleanse. Try to get one (or more) to join with you!

Then go to the grocery store and buy everything on the list. Go home. Get excited. I mean **REALLY EXCITED**.

Then you start juicing. Follow the procedure I've outlined for you. If you're new to juicing it may feel weird at first. Maybe you're unsure how to operate the juicer. Maybe you don't really know how long it will take to juice the produce. That's okay. By day three, you'll feel like a pro. By day seven, you'll wonder where the week went.

After the seven days, I want to hear about how it went!! Email me your stories. Share your struggles, your joys, your pains! We are SUPERheroes together in this cleanse so confide in me! Post your experience on your facebook page. Post your experience on MY facebook page. Tweet about it. Comment on my website blog. Tell your friends and family members. You get the idea.

To your SUPER RADIANT health,

Emyrald@PureRadiantSelf.com
PureRadiantSelf.com
Facebook.com/EmyraldSinclaire
PureRadiantSelf.com/2013/09/19/
superheros-unite/

Emyrald Sinclaire

ANOTHER BOOK BY EMYRALD SINCLAIRE....

THE 40 DAY JUICE CLEANSE!

- **Eliminate new toxins** from being introduced through food and drink.
- **Take the pressure off your digestive system**.
- Allow the body to use this "extra" energy to **rebalance your system and allow for deep healing**.
- Infuse your body with **safe, natural vitamins and minerals** in the most bio-available form almost instantly.
- **Boost your personal energy and vitality**!

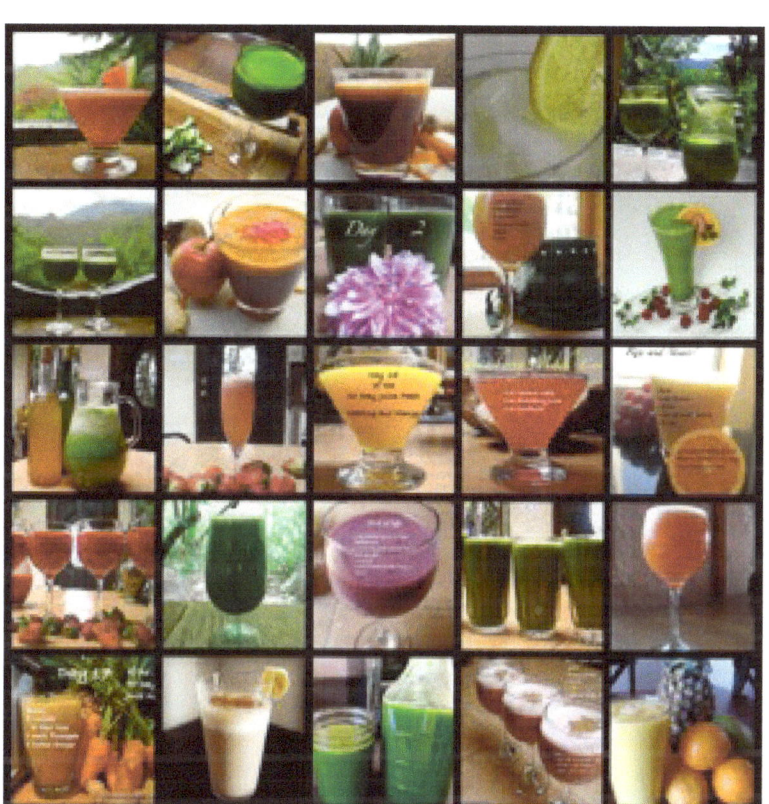

PureRadiantSelf.com/Juicing/40days/

E-BOOK:

scribd.com/doc/140822767/40-Days-of-Juicing-E-Book-by-Emyrald-Sinclaire

HARDCOPY:

www.createspace.com/4441420